DATE DUE

DEC 0 9 2004	

Springer Series: FOCUS ON WOMEN

Violet Franks, Ph.D., Series Editor
Confronting the major psychological, medical, and social issues of today and tomorrow. Focus on Women provides a wide range of books on the changing concerns of women.

Barbara Klug Redman, PhD, RN, FAAN, a nationally recognized researcher, administrator, and teacher, became the seventh dean of Wayne State University's College of Nursing September 1, 1998. Previously, Dr. Redman was dean of the School of Nursing at the University of Connecticut. She also has served as dean of nursing at the University of Colorado, associate dean at the University of Minnesota, and as executive director of the American Nurses Association and the American Association of Colleges of Nursing. Dr. Redman holds doctoral and master's degrees from the University of Minnesota and a bachelor's degree from South Dakota State University. She also has studied at Harvard Medical School, Johns Hopkins University, the University of Washington, Georgetown University, and George Washington University.

Dr. Redman received an Outstanding Achievement Award from the University of Minnesota, and Distinguished Service and Distinguished Alumnus Awards from South Dakota State University. In addition, she holds honorary doctoral degrees from Georgetown University and the University of Colorado.

Dr. Redman has taught at Johns Hopkins, University of Maryland, University of Minnesota and University of Washington. Her textbook, *The Practice of Patient Education,* is a mainstay in numerous nursing schools. Now in its eighth edition and used internationally, it focuses on how nurses teach patients to take care of themselves.

Women's Health Needs in Patient Education

Barbara K. Redman
PhD, RN, FAAN

Springer Series: Focus on Women

Copyright © 1999 by Springer Publishing Company, Inc.

Springer Publishing Company, Inc.
536 Broadway
New York, NY   10012-3955

Acquisitions Editor: Ruth Chasek
Production Editor: Pam Lankas
Cover design by James Scott-Lavino

99 00 01 02 03 / 5 4 3 2 1

Library of Congress Cataloging-in-Publication Data

Redman, Barbara Klug.
    Women's health needs in patient education / by Barbara K. Redman
        p.   cm. — (Springer series, focus on woman)
    Includes bibliographical references and index.
    ISBN 0-8261-1264-1 (hardcover)
    1. Patient education. 2. Women—Health and hygiene. I. Title.
II. Series: Springer series, focus on women (Unnumbered)
    [DNLM: 1. Women's Health. 2. Patient Education. 3. Primary
Prevention. WA 309 R318w 1999]
R727.4.R43   1999
615.5'071'082—DC21
DNLM/DLC
for Library of Congress   99-27854
                                                                  CIP

Printed in the United States of America

To Katherine Darlien Johnson (Katie)
For the next generation of women

Contents

Preface

Although I have long contributed to the field of patient education, in recent years I have been increasingly discomfited by the ethics of how it has traditionally been practiced, yet at the same time still believing that it is essential. Two years spent studying bioethics—first at the Kennedy Institute of Ethics at Georgetown University and then at Harvard Medical School—helped to clarify my concerns. Neither program included specific content on the ethics of patient education because bioethics has been focused on issues of concern to physicians. But basic ideas with which to approach my discomfort began to germinate.

This is not a basic text in patient education; many of those already exist. Neither does it address all possible education needed by women who are patients. Rather, it attempts to unmask the value assumptions hidden in the usual approach to patient education, from the perspective of one large group—women. It acknowledges that education can be yet an additional mechanism used by practitioners to control women and presents alternatives that I believe are more congruent with the needs of women. Patient education for women will continue to evolve for a long time to come.

List of Figures

List of Tables

CHAPTER ONE

The Gender Frame of Reference for Patient Education

T he field of women's health is finally developing with some rapidity, and perhaps the public's conscience has been awakened with evidence of historical and current inadequacies in the medical treatment of women. The focus of this book is the role of patient education in both hindering and facilitating that development. It includes identification of gaps in knowledge, skills, and perspectives that need to be developed to improve the health of women.

BACKGROUND

Chesney and Ozer (1995) have identified content areas in the study of women's health (see Figure 1.1). Some of these areas, such as those in the upper and right sections of the Figure, fall more clearly in the domain of patient education than do others. Many of these topics are covered in this book. Substance abuse, physical inactivity, violence prevention, and education are examples of topics that have been considered more in the domain of other psychosocial interventions, although smoking cessation is beginning to be incorporated into primary and maternity care.

A great deal of the patient-education literature relevant to women focuses on topics of reproductive health. Although no inference can be made that the preponderance of literature reflects educational services that are offered, it is reasonable to assume that if innovations were being developed in other areas of patient education for women, they would be more prevalent in the literature than they are. Even within categories identified in Figure 1.1, there are mismatches with the size of the bodies

1

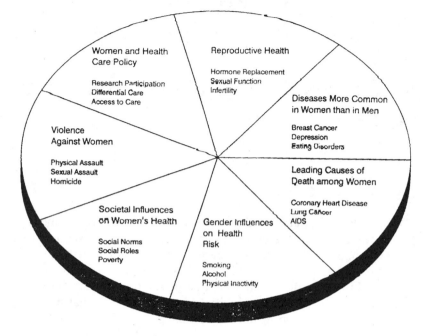

FIGURE 1.1   Content areas in the study of women's health.

From Chesney, M. A., & Ozer, E. M. (1995). Women and health: In search of a paradigm. *Woman's Health, 1,* 3–26. Copyright © 1995 Lawrence Erlbaum Associates. Reprinted by permission.

of literature. For example, although the leading cause of cancer death in women is lung cancer (Chesney & Ozer, 1995), many times more attention in the patient-education literature is paid to breast cancer.

A similar imbalance was found by Gannon, Stevens, and Stecker, (1997) in the content of articles published in three obstetrics and gynecology journals during the period of 1975–1993. The literature still heavily emphasized the reproductive nature of women rather than the health and well-being of nonpregnant and fertile women. The authors point out that a woman with two children spends 18 months pregnant and 30 years postmenopausal. The implicit message is that once a woman has fulfilled her biological role, she is of little interest to this specialty, as are women who are infertile or childless by choice.

Gannon et al. (1997) charge that these priorities do not reflect the reality of women's lives or their medical needs but rather are representative of sexist and outdated societal values and physicians' social and economic

interests. Feminists have charged that medical authority exercised with a clientele rendered vulnerable by oppressive gender roles has redefined normal developmental transitions such as menopause as diseases. According to this view, being a woman means being ill and is a source of weakness.

Historically, women have had their symptoms blamed on their reproductive systems; have undergone excessive, inappropriate, and experimental surgery; been overmedicated with tranquilizers; been excluded from research on which effective assessment and treatment depend (Candib, 1995); enjoyed less than equal access to important health care resources; and carried a burden disproportionate to that of men in the protection of fetal health. The next few years will see a revolution in both the philosophical and scientific bases for health care for women. Research related to gender will move well beyond its present state of ignoring it or infrequently noting differences between men and women. (Gender is the socially ascribed characteristics of females and males—their roles and appropriate behaviors, whereas sex is biological.)

Patient education is still affected by historic biases in health care about women and by the neglect of research on gender and sex differences in health. First, because most research on nonreproductive issues has been done on males, the information and skills included in patient-education programs may not be effective for women, and worse, may be misleading because patients believe they have been taught correct information. An example would be the presenting symptoms for myocardial infarction, which appear to differ for women.

Second, for many of the conditions that predominantly affect women, such as osteoporosis and urinary incontinence, patient-education programming has been scarce. Although neither condition is life threatening, both can be disabling, and women should have easy access to whatever is known about how to prevent or control them.

The third historical bias about gender roles has resulted in health policy that shifts care to the home, assumes that women will be the caregivers for families, and yet uses language of social neutrality to mask this fact. This social arrangement makes it important for women to develop a broad range of skill in health. Fourth, reproductive roles as they are construed today make women high consumers of contraceptive, fertility, and genetic services. Each of these services requires education first on choice and decisions, and then on how to use these services with an appropriate balance of concern for the women and for the family unit.

Practitioners must learn how to construct more positive models of care for women such as empowerment and options for joint decision making. Norm redefinition is also necessary, as in the example of aging. For example, male norms imply that older, sicker, and widowed women are a societal problem. Rather, the focus should be on women's ability to survive and on the strength of their networks in old age.

Worse yet are health care approaches and the resulting educational messages that make women responsible for men's behavior. An example is the use of condoms as the primary means for HIV prevention. Many women do not have the power to negotiate use of condoms by their partners and then are left with no means of protection and no choice in avoiding exposure.

What is known about gender suggests that instructional approaches to women might differ. In addition, the psychometric characteristics of tools used to assess learning needs or measure outcomes from patient education may not have been tested for validity across gender, race, or class. Yet the use of gender-sensitive measurement tools holds great promise in promoting healthy outcomes for women.

Gender affects employment, income, occupation, and empowerment, all of which affect health states through their impact on available time for self-care, role behavior in perceiving and presenting symptoms, and in negotiating treatment (Kunkel, 1996). Women's choices and their ability to deal with health issues have been affected by public policies, the scientific research that sometimes informs them, and the press, which serves a large educational role.

SOCIAL POLICY

A number of policies related to health and disability have been constructed, knowingly or not, to give men an advantage over women. Three examples are instructive. First, the acute care bias in Medicare coverage corresponds to a male pattern of illness and is a particular disadvantage to older, low-income and minority women, who bear a disproportionate share of chronic illnesses (Dressel, Minkler, & Yen, 1997). Second, because public policy neglects caring work as a societal responsibility, women bear the costs of this work. Because most women do caring work at one or more times during their lifetimes, the economic disadvantage from it accumulates for them, contributing (along with other social policies such as lack of equal pay) to poverty in their later years (Meyer, 1997). The technological focus on health care increases the pressure on family caregiving (read mother, daughter, and wife).

Finally, those disabilities that are most common in males such as spinal-cord injuries, are better supported through public funds for treatment, rehabilitation, and wheelchair access. In other words, certain kinds of illnesses and disabilities have been privileged within Western social and biomedical decision making. This response does not reflect the actual population demographics of disability and is inconsistent with notions of distributive social justice (Thorne, McCormick, & Carty, 1997).

SCIENTIFIC THOUGHT AND RESEARCH

It appears that there are significant and widespread differences in the normal physiology of men and women and in the way disease is expressed in each of the two genders (Legato, 1997). Many of these differences are not yet well understood.

Even today, only a quarter of studies with female and male subjects reported any data analysis by gender. Differential responses of women and men to intervention and treatment protocols are still not routinely discussed in the recommendations of published studies (Charney & Morgan, 1996).

Candib (1995) suggests that medical thought is structured on family life-cycle theory. This theory holds empty or negative imagery about postmenopausal women, implying an end to meaningful development with the end of the reproductive phase of life. Western physicians have considered women to be far more troubled by menopausal symptoms than women themselves report. Life-cycle theory also sees paid employment for women as an additional stress in family life.

Women's longevity is seen as creating a surplus of women who express more symptoms than do men and "overuse" health services. In research, it is widowhood and not social network strength that is used as a variable in the analysis of service use and institutionalization (Gibson, 1996).

THE PRESS AS EDUCATOR

The press has also played a role in shaping attitudes about women's health. A study of how cancer has historically been portrayed in the press (Reagan, 1997) found a pattern of attributing modesty toward pelvic exams as a factor in causing cancer deaths in women. Women's breast cancer has been portrayed as a penalty for not having children and nursing them. Yet no one suggested women might be better off by avoiding sex with men to decrease the odds of cervical cancer or that lesbian relationships were also protective. Finally, adult women were considered responsible for monitoring and detecting signs and symptoms of cancer in family members and blamed if they failed (Reagan, 1997).

Debates on drug addiction and fetal harm have indicated that women alone bear the burden and blame for production of "crack babies." It was assumed that men not rendered infertile by their toxic exposures were immune from any other form of reproductive risk, such as genetic damage. Since at least the late 1980s, however, studies have shown a clear link between paternal exposure to drugs, alcohol, smoking, environmental and occupational toxins, and fetal health problems, yet men have been spared the blame (Daniels, 1997).

Labor policies regarding occupational hazards and labels on liquor and cigarettes have assumed that women are the only vulnerable individuals and thus the primary source of fetal harm. Public health warnings carried in the press for men focus on behaviors that cause harm to themselves and for women focus exclusively on their harm to others (the fetus). Studies of women and drug abuse, on which public health warnings are based, still don't control for their occupational exposure, whereas studies of birth hazards related to occupational risks of soldiers do not consider their potential drug abuse (Daniels, 1997).

A common theme in debates and newspaper coverage over abortion, working mothers, or pregnancy and addiction, concerns women's failure to subordinate their own interests to the needs of born and unborn children (Daniels, 1997).

A REVISED PATIENT EDUCATION FOR WOMEN

Traditionally, medicine has defined problems as requiring changes in the person to fit an unquestioned social order. Deficit-oriented diagnoses; interventions that are reactive instead of proactive; and a focus on individuals, families, and small groups rather than on systems, are still typical (Prilleltensky, 1997).

A new set of ethical standards should undergird how knowledge is used in relationships with patients. The following should be seen as unethical:

- minimizing a client's autonomy by excluding her from decision-making processes,
- stigmatizing individuals with labels that describe only their deficits,
- defining problems exclusively in individual terms and neglecting to consider social injustices, and
- assuming to know what is best for clients (Prilleltensky, 1997).

The chapters that follow provide suggestions for helping women learn skills in specific areas of health and for which information is missing or biased, they also provide a basis for understanding the scope of the work that remains to be accomplished. What can be done to make patient education for women a more informed, less biased endeavor?

Mechanic (1997) notes that at any point in time the practice of medicine is a mixture of theories at varying levels of confirmation and a variety of social judgments and prejudices. Physician roles substantially transcend the corpus of medical knowledge, and both patients and societies demand that doctors provide assistance even when knowledge is limited. This means that there are enormous opportunities for value judgments to be played out under the guise of clinical determinations. Rozin (1997) notes that health issues typically have a moral component, and moralization of health issues is more likely for stigmatized or marginalized groups, which women have traditionally been.

The nature of helping and of the research being developed to further inform it necessarily involve values. These must be as positive for women as they have been for men and must support their diversity. Through new scientific findings and partnerships with patients, patient education should become more efficacious than it has been and a more positive force in our patients' lives.

REFERENCES

Candib, L. M. (1995). *Medicine and the family.* New York: Basic Books.

Charney, P., & Morgan, C. (1996). Do treatment recommendations reported in the research literature consider differences between women and men? *Journal of Women's Health 5,* 579–584.

Chesney, M. A., & Ozer, E. M. (1995). Women and health: In search of a paradigm. *Women's Health, 1,* 3–26.

Daniels, C. R. (1997). Between fathers and fetuses: The social construction of male reproduction and the politics of fetal harm. *Signs: Journal of Women in Culture and Society, 22,* 579–616.

Dressel, P., Minkler, M., & Yen, I. (1997). Gender, race, class, and aging: Advances and opportunities. *International Journal of Health Services, 27,* 579–600.

Gannon, L., Stevens, J., & Stecker, T. (1997). A content analysis of obstetrics and gynecology scholarship: Implications for women's health. *Women & Health, 26,* 41–55.

Gibson, D. (1996). Broken down by age and gender. *Gender and Society, 10,* 433–448.

Kunkel, S. R. (1996). Why gender matters: Being female is not the same as being male. *American Journal of Preventive Medicine, 12,* 294–295.

Legato, M. J. (1997). Gender-specific physiology: How real is it? How important is it? *International Journal of Fertility, 42,* 19–29.

Mechanic, D. (1997). The social context of health and disease and choices among health interventions. In A. Brandt & P. Rozin (Eds.), *Morality and health.* New York: Routledge.

Meyer, M. H. (1997). Toward a structural, life course agenda for reducing insecurity among women as they age. *Gerontologist, 37,* 833–834.

Prilleltensky, I. (1997). Values, assumptions and practices. *American Psychologist, 52,* 517–535.

Reagan, L. J. (1997). Engendering the dread disease: Women, men and cancer. *American Journal of Public Health, 87,* 1779–1787.

Rozin, P. (1997). Moralization. In A. Brandt & P. Rozin (Eds.), *Morality and health.* New York: Routledge.

Thorne, S., McCormick, J., & Carty, E. (1997). Deconstructing the gender neutrality of chronic illness and disability. *Health Care for Women International, 18,* 1–16.

CHAPTER TWO

Cardiovascular Education

PATTERNS OF DIFFERENCE

Across the entire lifetime, cardiovascular disease (CVD) is slightly more common as a cause of mortality in women than in men. The increase with age lags behind the male-associated increase by 10 to 15 years with African American women more susceptible to CVD than Caucasian women. Angina pectoris is an earlier and more common presentation of the arteriosclerotic process in women than in men. Frank myocardial infarction (MI) in women has more unfavorable consequences than in men, with sudden death more frequent. Operative procedures for CVD show a greater short-and long-term morbidity and mortality in women than in men (Knopp, 1998). Cardiovascular anatomy and physiology as it differs in women and men may be found in Table 2.1 (Romeo, 1995).

Despite the fact that heart disease is the leading cause of death and disability for women, many women do not understand that fact, patterns of care have not adapted to women's needs, and standard patient education has not incorporated their different experiences. By now, the pattern is clear. Both technologies and drugs used with heart disease and hypertension were developed and tested (frequently with public funding) primarily on Whites and males. In a study of California hospital discharges in 1989 and 1990, Giacomini (1996) found that women received a number of procedures including coronary artery bypass grafts (CABGs) and percutaneous transluminal coronary angioplasty (PTCA) less frequently than did men. Because the study controlled for insurance status as well as admission to hospitals providing the procedures, the findings could not easily be explained as a two-tiered delivery system. Whether the differences represented undertreatment or overtreatment for particular groups could not be determined.

Women are at greater risk of experiencing adverse reactions from cardiovascular drugs as differential doses and uses for females for

TABLE 2.1   Women's Cardiovascular Physiology

Cardiovascular anatomy and physiology characteristics of women, which are different from men include:

• Smaller stature
• Smaller heart
• Smaller coronary vessels
• Single vessel disease more prevalent
• More vasospasm
• More atypical chest pain
• More variant angina
• Variable response to noninvasive tests
• Shorter PR and QRS intervals
• Smaller amplitude of R, S, and T across the precordium
• Lower left ventricular end-diastolic pressure
• Lower left ventricular volume
• Higher resting ejection fraction
• No increase in ejection fraction with exercise
• First manifestation of CVD usually angina
• Signs and symptoms of CVD trail men by 10–20 years
• Higher first-year mortality after MI
• Additional risk factors of menopause, oral contraceptive use and employment-role conflict

Used with permission from K. C. Romeo: "The Female Heart: Physiological Aspects of Cardiovascular Disease in Women," *Dimensions of Critical Care Nursing, 14*(4), 170, © Springhouse Corporation.

commonly prescribed cardiac drugs have rarely been studied. This is particularly true for diuretics and antilipemics. Research has usually focused on differences based on race and age with exclusion of gender (Morgan, Colling, & Fye, 1996). Although they could benefit as much as men, women are less frequently referred to cardiac rehabilitation programs and fewer complete the programs. Indeed, the programs themselves have changed little since they were first developed for men in the 1960s (Moore, 1996a).

Conventional explanations for these patterns include: (a) different patient preferences, (b) barriers to access, (c) provider attitudes toward women sometimes manifested in clinical eligibility differences and communication patterns about treatment options, and (d) lack of clarity about whether these services are overused in men or underused in women because of a lack of clinical trials, including enough women and minorities to yield adequate evidence of different effectiveness in different demographic groups. Where this evidence is lacking, clinicians may be reluctant to embark on aggressive interventions in patients from unstudied groups. The design of technologies may also be partly responsible for their differential allocation (Giacomini, 1996).

If patient preferences differ by gender, they could result from the way providers communicate treatment options, negative patient experiences elsewhere in the health care system, patient education level especially with regard to the merits of high-technology medicine, or patients' personal expenses not being covered by insurance. Yet, the patient-preference theory for differential treatment of men and women inadequately explains the systematic usage differences that prevail across a number of procedures that almost entirely favor Whites and men (Giacomini, 1996).

If these patterns are further verified, educational programs serving women with heart disease should arm them with the knowledge they need to assure that they demand the treatment that is best for them. Such a goal would be difficult to incorporate into current patient-education programs because their role has traditionally been to assist patients to comply with current medical treatment, not challenge it.

The differences between men and women manifest themselves at every stage of disease and treatment. In prevention, women with mild to moderate hypertension were less likely to be given relevant counseling even though nearly all had at least one modifiable risk factor. Men were significantly more likely to be advised to adopt a low-cholesterol diet, lose weight, stop smoking, decrease alcohol intake, or exercise more (Foss et al., 1996). Nearly 60% of women who reported regular medical checkups also reported that their physicians never spoke with them about heart disease or recommended cholesterol checks. These women believed that they were unlikely to have a heart attack at some point in their lives. It can be concluded that many women are either not counseled at all or are inadequately counseled about their susceptibility to cardiovascular disease (Legato, Padus, & Slaughter, 1997).

Differences also occur at the time symptoms are noted. Women on average took an hour longer to present for medical care for symptoms of acute myocardial infarction (AMI). History of cardiac disease had no discernible effect on the occurrence of prolonged delay (Gurwitz et al., 1997; Morgan et al., 1996). Although aware of their symptoms as abnormal, the women believed that heart disease affected primarily men and that their symptoms did not fit the pattern for AMI. Delays of this sort are serious because the opportunity for management of dysrhythmias and early intervention with thrombolytic agents is lost. These agents can reestablish perfusion, limit infarct size, preserve left ventricular function, and reduce the number of deaths (Dempsey, Dracup, & Moser, 1995). Nausea and dyspnea are more frequent complaints of females than the vise-like chest pain or radiating arm pain that commonly heralds AMI in men, and the distribution of women's pain may not be simply in the substernal area but also in the upper abdomen, shoulder, or neck (Legato et al., 1997).

No proven method is currently available for for educating patients to hasten their presentations for care in response to symptoms suggestive of AMI. Nevertheless, a better understanding of the role of women's knowledge and symptom interpretation will aid in developing educational interventions specifically targeted at them (Gurwitz et al., 1997). This should include educational programs to increase the awareness of persons with established cardiac risk factors of the need for prompt response to symptoms.

More than a quarter of individuals undergoing CABG are women. They present at an older age and with more symptoms and comorbidity than do men. Many of their recovery experiences are not addressed in traditional CABG discharge teaching. These include sharp, numb, burning, heavy or tingling sensations in the breasts, sometimes described as related to the incision and lasting for weeks. The women were not prepared for these sensations and did not know how to manage them (Moore, 1996b). Instead of following guidelines for activity resumption, women used family and home responsibilities and level of fatigue to guide their activity (Hawthorne, 1994). Many women show greater anxiety and depression post AMI or CABG than do men, thus indicating a need for interventions that address psychological states and affective recovery from coronary events (Low, 1993).

Women in Hawthorne's study (1994) had major difficulty in communicating with predominantly male physicians who were presumed to have higher status and power. The passivity and deference consistently displayed by women patients is thought to lessen the amount of critical information provided by and to patients, thereby seriously diminishing the validity of clinical assessments and treatment plans for women and their instruction in self-care.

Post-CABG, women are more at risk for adverse outcomes and yet have the least recovery support because they are older and live alone (Moore, 1996b). They have poorer outcomes from CABG, less relief of symptoms, and higher mortality rates (Cronin, Logsdon, & Miracle, 1997). Female gender has been associated with increased likelihood of rehospitalization. In various studies, increasing hospitalization in patients with AMI has been associated with less cardiac lifestyle knowledge, a higher level of emotional distress, and failed social-support systems, among other factors. Other studies have shown that nurse-directed interventions can decrease hospital readmission for heart failure by half (Maynard, Every, & Weaver, 1997).

Only a small percentage of women who experience cardiac events are referred to formal cardiac rehabilitation programs and drop out of such programs at a higher rate then do their male counterparts. Data on rehabilitative outcomes for women are limited, and most guidelines for reha-bilitation interventions are derived from studies of men. Women eligible for cardiac rehabilitation programs are already different from men in being older; more likely to be hypertensive, diabetic and obese; and exhibiting poorer functional status with more shortness of breath, less activity, and more chronic illness. Congruent with this situation, women in cardiac rehabilitation programs had more concerns about pain and fatigue while exercising. In addition, they desired more social interaction during the exercise sessions and more emotional support from staff members about all dimensions of cardiac recovery. Social support has been shown to be a more important predictor of exercise participation for women than men (Moore, 1996b; Moore & Kramer, 1996).

For women, a rehabilitation center that offers a place to talk may be just as critical to recovery as is an exercise gym because women tend to use a relational way of coping. Having a place to ask questions and to really understand the meaning of lifestyle changes, coupled with inter-personal support, can make a major difference in women following the rehabilitation regimen (Arnold, 1997). Because the few intervention stud-ies that address psychosocial issues after a cardiac event have not exam-ined the experience of women, the type of psychosocial rehabilitation that might be beneficial to women is not known (Fleury & Cameron-Go, 1997). At the conclusion of cardiac rehabilitation programs, men report better quality of life, less chest pain and shortness of breath, and greater energy (Deshotels, Planchock, & Prevost, 1995).

Current cardiac rehabilitation program design and operational features are perceived by some women studied as not meeting their needs (Moore, 1996a). Focus groups showed that women disliked programs with limited exercise choices and emotional support. They liked the outcomes of confi-dence in the ability to resume activities of daily living, feeling better, im-proved nutrition knowledge and skills from hands-on teaching, and the availability of a support group. Because women believe they are not receiv-ing full benefits, cardiac rehabilitation programs should be redesigned to incorporate elements that would engage them and create positive outcomes.

HYPERTENSION

Approximately one quarter of the population of the industrialized world has hypertension, with almost 60% of these being women. Through middle age, the prevalence of hypertension is higher among men than women; it then reverses. In younger women, pregnancy can induce hypertension as can oral-contraceptive use.

Until recently, investigators assumed that no gender-specific differences existed in diagnosis, prognosis, and treatment of hypertension. Because women have been underrepresented in clinical trials and trials did not address gender differences, guidelines for care are generally not differentiated by sex. The dosage and schedule of therapy for most drugs were designed for men despite the potential for different effects in women who differ in body size, percentage of body fat, and fat distribution. Although no therapies have been shown to be ineffective in women, firm conclusions of optimal drug choices for women cannot be drawn (Hayes & Taler, 1998).

Little is known about the effects of menopause or the interaction between hormone replacement therapy (HRT) and different antihypertensive agents. Although long recognized in men, sexual dysfunction induced by antihypertensive therapy is largely ignored in women, and study questions have not been specific to problems women commonly experience. In general, women are more likely to be aware of their blood pressure, more likely to be receiving treatment, and if so more likely to have achieved blood pressure control (Hayes & Taler, 1998; Schenck-Gustafsson, 1996).

So although evidence shows that gender differences in hypertension exist, definitive studies from which to draw firm conclusions regarding the extent and importance of these differences are lacking (Hayes & Taler, 1998). Perhaps patient-education programs should alert women patients to the limitations of the knowledge that undergirds their treatment and how to determine if treatment is not as effective as it might be.

MITRAL VALVE PROLAPSE

Mitral valve prolapse (MVP) is systolic billowing of the valve's posterior leaflets into the atrium, possibly involving elongated chordae tendinae and papillary muscle dysfunction. Some cases are accompanied by autonomic dysfunction and are labelled MVP syndrome (MVPS). Incidence is as high as 10%, with women being affected twice as often as men. MVP is believed to be inherited, with a greater expression of the MVP gene in women (Alpert, Sabik, & Cosgrove, 1998; McGrath, 1997; Scordo, 1997).

Fifty percent of women with MVP report fatigue, palpitations, and a forceful pounding heart beat, atypical chest pain that sometimes mimics angina, dyspnea, exercise intolerance, dizziness with postural change problems sleeping, anxiety, and/or panic attacks. There is no correlation between symptoms and the degree of prolapse, and it is not unusual for the symptoms to disappear spontaneously for months or years and reappear again. Natural-history studies show that most individuals with MVPS have a relatively benign prognosis and rarely require valve replacement.

The disorder is rarely explained to women who suffer from it. Some people mistakenly envision holes in the valve when told they have a leaky valve. Pictures or models of the heart will help, as will an analogy to a parachute opening in explaining billowing of the valve. Many patients mistakenly believe their chest pain is the prelude to a MI.

Self-care measures to alleviate or control the common symptoms can be taught. To guard against bacterial endocarditis, patients must learn to request antibiotic prophylaxis before surgery and invasive dental or oral procedures. Caffeine is to be avoided. Regular cardiovascular exercise has been shown to decrease the frequency and intensity of MVPS symptoms. Because patients may be afraid that something dreadful will happen to them when they exercise, a cardiac rehabilitation unit provides a safe environment and helps to alleviate fears. Patients can be taught that sometimes a change of position relieves chest pain. Some patients with MVPS are quite sensitive to volume depletion and should be advised to drink a minimum of eight glasses of water per day. Support groups are reported to be available (Hayes & Taler, 1998; McGrath, 1997; Scordo, 1998). A great need to develop and make available programs to educate patients with MPVS and their families exists. An excellent book on MVPS for patients has been authored by Scordo (1994).

PREVENTION OF CARDIOVASCULAR DISEASE

Some work has been done to understand the special needs of women of color to prevent cardio-vascular disease. Of special concern is the fact that Black and Mexican American women have higher levels of cardiovascular risk factors than do White women of comparable age and socioeconomic status (SES). Within each of the ethnic groups, women of low SES tend to have higher levels of risk factors. Although past preventive efforts have been effective in reaching White women and those of higher

SES, they have been less effective in reaching minority women and those of lower SES. Health systems need effective protocols to reach these women, who often experience differential access to services because of cost barriers, unavailability of health insurance, and discrimination in health care (Winkleby, Kraemer, Ahn, & Varady, 1998).

Prevention education is also important for first-degree relatives of female patients with premature coronary heart disease (CHD). These individuals are at greater risk for earlier disease than if the proband is a male patient. Allen and Blumenthal (1998) examined apparently healthy offspring of women with documented premature CHD (as evidenced by CABG or AMI before age 60) and found a high proportion overweight with high prevalence of central obesity, half with total and low-density lipoprotein cholesterol levels above recommended levels, 31% who were currently smokers, and 56% exercising fewer than three times a week. Many had multiple risk factors. The incidence of obesity and diabetes was especially high in female offspring.

Most did not perceive themselves to be at risk for CHD, in part because they believed they did not take after that side of the family or had a lifestyle different from that of the affected relative. Because familial-clustered CHD accounts for 55%–60% of total documented coronary disease before age 60 and many of these risk factors are modifiable, individuals with a family history of premature CHD should be targeted for education and screening (Allen & Blumenthal, 1998).

IMPLICATIONS FOR PATIENT-EDUCATION PROGRAMS

A common psychosocial theme expressed by women with cardiovascular heart disease is the feeling of not being heard. At a loss as to how to understand and cope with a new constellation of feelings not easily understood or supported by those in their environment including their physicians, these women unnecessary flounder and can be further incapacitated by their negative feelings (Arnold, 1997).

Although it may not be necessary to construct gender-specific programs, attention to the gender differences outlined previously is important. Some examples of teaching approaches specifically developed for women with cardiovascular disease follow.

Preparatory sensory information is recommended for adults about to undergo threatening procedures as this information helps them know what to expect, how to cope more effectively, and experience less distress. Previous studies have shown that patients so prepared report less anxiety, require less medication, and are more satisfied with their care than are patients who receive no preparatory intervention or one based only on a description of the procedure.

For preparatory sensory information to be most effective in helping patients, it must include words and phrases that describe the subjective experiences of persons who have already undergone the procedure, describing what the person saw, heard, felt, smelled, and tasted at times during the procedure. Cason and Landis (1995) have studied women's sensory experiences during cardiac catheterization. Their findings may be found in Table 2.2. If verified with a larger and diverse group of women, this information can be used in teaching programs.

Allen (1996) tested a nurse-directed risk-factor modification program in women after coronary artery bypass surgery. Based on a self-efficacy (SE) model (Table 2.3), this intervention focuses on the means by which SE has been shown to develop (performance accomplishment, vicarious experience or the observance of others performing the behavior and evaluating the consequences, physiological arousal and feedback, and the physical feelings that accompany performance of the activity). This behaviorally oriented self-help program involved use of workbook and videotapes, smoking-cessation counseling and individualized dietary and exercise instruction based on the patient's progress toward mutually established goals. These elements were delivered economically in a short in-hospital session followed by a single home visit and subsequent telephone-based contact.

The intervention proved more effective than usual medical care in reducing the dietary intake of fat and saturated fat, and increasing smoking cessation. Although self-efficacy theory is broadly applicable across many populations, Allen's model notes the importance of using other female patients who have had the same surgery as teaching models.

Ashton's (1997) review of studies on teaching and learning in cardiac disease published in the early 1990s shows that they also followed the pattern of including many more men than women in their study samples. In addition, none of this research addressed gender differences. Ashton's own research showed that following AMI, both men and women ranked risk factors and medications as most important to learn.

A randomized controlled trial to evaluate an intervention to enhance self-management of heart disease by older individuals did study effects by gender. Through these disease self-management programs, patients learn to carry out at home the recommendations of their clinicians and manage the physical and psychosocial impairment that disease can en-

TABLE 2.2   Cardiac Catheterization Procedural Phases and Associated Sensations—The Experiences of 14 Women

Phase	Sensations*
Phase 1	
Patient placed on table, connected to cardiac monitor undressed, and partially covered with a cloth.	
Intravenous vein sited or checked for patency.	
Pulse oximeter applied.	
Groin area swabbed with betadine.†	Coldness
Phase 2	
Sterile drapes lowered.	
Pressure transducer, equipment, and contrast medium prepared.	
Sedation administered. Physician locates pulse in right groin.	
Needle inserted and groin area numbed with xylocaine.	Stick, stinging, burning
Phase 3	
Physician makes small incision in groin and enlarges it with hemostats.	
Physician palpates artery and inserts needle into artery.	Pressure in groin
Phase 4	
Guidewire and dilator-sheath assembly inserted into artery.	
Dilator removed.	Pressure, pulling in groin
Phase 5	
Guidewire removed blood aspirated into sheath to clear air.	
Sheath flushed with saline.	
Catheter inserted and visualized on fluoroscope.	
Phase 6	
Monitor observed for heart pressures; pressures recorded.	
Dye injected mechanically.‡	Warm, hot, burning feelings
Dye transit observed on fluoroscopy.	Whole body/all over/top to toe/ head to bottom
	Chest/throat
	Feeling of having urinated on oneself
Phase 7	
Guidewire reinserted, catheter removed.	
Second catheter inserted.	
Catheter insertion visualized on fluoroscopy.	
Dye injected by hand.	
Dye transit observed on fluoroscopy.	No response

(continued)

TABLE 2.2   (Continued)

Phase	Sensations*
Phase 8 Guidewire reinserted, catheter removed. Third catheter inserted. Catheter insertion visualized on fluoroscopy. Dye injected by hand. Dye transit observed on fluoroscopy. Catheter and guidewire removed. Sheath removed and occlusive pressure applied to groin.	Pressure/discomfort in leg
Phase 9 Occlusive pressure maintained for 15–20 min. Benzoin spray and pressure dressing applied, patient placed on hospital bed or stretcher and returned to room or holding area.	Cold spray

*Only sensations reported by 40% or more of women are listed. †Patient's groin was washed and shaved before patient arrived in cardiac catheterization laboratory. ‡Iovorsol (74%) was the contrast medium for all subjects.

From Cason, Carolyn L., and Landis, Marilyn. (1995). Women's sensory experiences during cardiac catheterization. *Cardiovascular Nursing 31*(5): 33–36. Reprinted by permission of the American Heart Association.

gender in daily life. On the basis of the findings, Clark et al. (1997) suggest separate interventions for men and women. The intervention must be designed to address the higher number and greater intensity of symptoms women experienced and the greater negative impact of the illness on their physical functioning.

Well-validated measurement tools are important for patient assessment and evaluation of patient-education outcomes. Several tools for cardiovascular patient education may be found in Redman (1998). No instrument with well-established norms for women or one specially designed to reflect the differences for women as outlined in this chapter, could be located.

SUMMARY

Evidence of women's special needs in cardiovascular patient education is accumulating. Although education could be a significant part of inter-

TABLE 2.3   **Application of the Self-Efficacy Model in the Development of Special Interventions**

Components of self-efficacy model	Related special intervention strategies
Performance accomplishments	Set small individualized goals with the patient in a series of behaviors that can be consecutively mastered so she experiences success.
	Rehearse desired behaviors with the nurse.
	Have patient keep a log of activities and diet to promote self-reinforcement.
Verbal persuasion	Provide strong verbal encouragement of relative progress.
	Attribute accomplishments to patient's own abilities.
	Use an experienced intervention nurse who is a highly credible source.
	Incorporate significant others into the intervention to increase their support and reinforcement of behaviors.
Physiological arousal	Help interpret symptoms accurately and promote relaxation training to decrease anxiety and feelings of physical inefficacy.
Vicarious experience	Draw attention to relative progress of other female CABS patients of similar age through female model in videotape.
Cognitive appraisal	Provide counseling sessions to help patient process information, solve problems, and generalize self-efficacy.

From Allen, Jerilyn K. (1996). Coronary risk factor modification in women after coronary artery bypass surgery. *Nursing Research, 45,* 260–265. Copyright © 1996 by Lippincott, Williams & Wilkins. Reprinted by permission.

ventions to meet many of these needs, there is little in the literature that indicates it has been developed and is available. Women are further disadvantaged when providers do not acknowledge their symptoms and experiences that differ from the male norm. Educational programming for women with cardiovascular disease should be a high priority with careful evaluation of what it contributes. Given historic lack of access by women to cardiovascular treatment and especially to treatment known to be efficacious for their sex, advocacy/empowerment educational pro-

grams that teach women how to evaluate their care and demand efficacious treatment are also important.

REFERENCES

Allen, J. K. (1996). Coronary risk factor modification in women after coronary
artery bypass surgery. *Nursing Research, 45,* 260–265.
Allen, J. K., & Blumenthal, R. S. (1998). Risk factors in the offspring of
women with premature coronary heart disease. *American Heart Journal,
135,* 428–434.
Alpert, J. S., Sabik, J., & Cosgross, D. M. (1998). Mitral valve disease. In E.
J. Topol (Ed.). *Textbook of cardiovascular medicine.* Philadelphia: Lippin-
cott-Raven.
Arnold, E. (1997). The stress connection; women and coronary heart disease.
Critical Care Nursing Clinics of North America, 9, 565–575.
Ashton, K. C. (1997). Perceived learning needs of men and women after my-
ocardial infarction. *Journal of Cardiovascular Nursing, 12,* 93–100.
Cason, C. L., & Landis, M. (1995). Women's sensory experiences during car-
diac catheterization. *Cardiovascular Nursing 31,* 33–36.
Clark, N. M., Janz., N. K., Dodge, J. A., Schork, M. A., Wheeler, J. R. C.,
Liang, J., Keteyian, S. L., & Santinga, J. T. (1997). Self-management of
heart disease by older adults. *Research on Aging, 19,* 362–382.
Cronin, S. N., Logsdon, C., & Miracle, V. (1997). Psychosocial and functional
outcomes in women after coronary artery bypass surgery. *Critical Care Nurse,
17(2),* 19–24.
Dempsey, S. J., Dracup, K., & Moser, D. K. (1995). Women's decision to seek
care for symptoms of acute myocardial infarction. *Heart & Lung, 24,* 444–
456.
Deshotels, A., Planchock, N., Dech, A., & Prevost, S. (1995). Gender differences in perceptions of quality of life in cardiac rehabilitation patients. *Journal
of Cardiopulmonary Rehabilitation 15,* 143–148.
Fleury, J., & Cameron-Go, K. (1997). Women's rehabilitation and recovery.
Critical Care Nursing Clinics of North America, 9, 577–587.
Foss, F. A., Dickinson, E., Hills, N., Thomson, A., Wilson, V., & Ebrahim, S.
(1996). Missed opportunities for the prevention of cardiovascular disease
among British hypertensives in primary care. *British Journal of General
Practice, 46,* 571–575.
Giacomini, M. K. (1996). Gender and ethnic differences in hospital-based pro-

cedure utilization in California. *Archives of Internal Medicine, 156,* 1217–1224.

Gurwitz, J. H., McLaughlin, T. S., Willison, D. J., Quadagnoli, E., Hauptman, P. J., Gao, X., & Soumerai, S. B. (1997). Delayed hospital presentation in patients who have had acute myocardial infarction. *Annals of Internal Medicine, 126,* 593–599.

Hawthorne, M. H. (1994). Gender differences in recovery after coronary artery surgery. *Image, 26,* 75–80.

Hayes, S. N. & Taler, S. J. (1998). Hypertension in women: current understanding of gender differences. *Mayo Clinic Proceedings, 73,* 157–165.

Knopp, R. H. (1998). Estrogen, female gender, and heart disease. In E. J. Topol (Ed.), *Textbook of cardiovascular medicine.* Philadelphia: Lippincott-Raven.

Legato, M. J., Padus, E., & Slaughter, E. (1997). Women's perceptions of their general health, with special reference to their risk of coronary artery disease: Results of a national telephone survey. *Journal of Women's Health, 6,* 189–198.

Low, K. G. (1993). Recovery from myocardial infarction and coronary artery bypass surgery in women: Psychosocial factors. *Journal of Women's Health, 2,* 133–139.

Maynard, C., Every, N. R., & Weaver, W. D. (1997). Factors associated with rehospitalization in patients with acute myocardial infarction. *American Journal of Cardiology, 80,* 777–779.

McGrath, D. (1997). Mitral valve prolapse. *American Journal of Nursing, 97(5),* 40–41.

Moore, S. M. (1996a). Women's views of cardiac rehabilitation programs. *Journal of Cardiopulmonary Rehabilitation, 16,* 123–129.

Moore, S. M. (1996b). CABG discharge information. *Clinical Nursing Research, 5,* 97–104.

Moore, S. M., & Kramer, F. M. (1996). Women's and men's preferences for cardiac rehabilitation program features. *Journal of Cardiopulmonary Rehabilitation, 16,* 163–168.

Morgan, N. A., Colling, C. L., & Fye, C. L. (1996). Cardiovascular diseases in women: an equal opportunity killer. *Journal of the American Pharmaceutical Association, NS36,* 360–369.

Redman, B. K. (1998). *Measurement tools in patient education.* New York: Springer Publishing Co.

Romeo, K. C. (1995). The female heart: physiological aspects of cardiovascular disease in women. *Dimensions of Critical Care Nursing, 14,* 170–177.

Schenck-Gustafsson, K. (1996). Risk factors for cardiovascular disease in women: assessment and management. *European Heart Journal, 17(Suppl. D),* 2–8.

Scordo, K. A. B. (1998). Mitral valve prolapse syndrome: Interventions for symptom control. *Dimensions of Critical Care Nursing, 17,* 177–186.

Scordo, K. A. B. (1997). Mitral valve prolapse syndrome. *Critical Care Nursing Clinics of North America, 9,* 555–564.

Scordo, K. A. (1994). *Taking control: Living with mitral valve prolapse syndrome.* Columbia, SC: Camden House.

Winkelby, M. A., Kraemer, H. C., Ahn, D. K., & Varady, A. N. (1998). Ethnic and socioeconomic differences in cardiovascular disease risk factors. *Journal of the American Medical Association, 280,* 356–362.

CHAPTER THREE

Gynecologic, Genitourinary, and Reproductive Patient Education

Given the historic focus on women's reproductive functions to the exclusion of other functions, one might expect the full development of patient education on gynecologic, genitourinary, and reproductive topics. On the other hand, many of these areas are of most relevance to the woman experiencing them and not of broader use to society in assuring her reproductive function. In each of these topics (menarche, reproductive education, menopause and associated risk for osteoporosis, and urinary incontinence)—education has been relatively unavailable, and messages have been heavily medically oriented. Feminists have suggested broader views.

MENARCHE AND MENSTRUATION

One would presume that understanding of bodily changes surrounding menarche and of menstruation itself would be important for self-care and for reproductive care. Studies of young girls show that their understanding of these subjects is frequently faulty. Sixth grade girls were found not to understand how the egg, blood, and uterus were interrelated. Origin of menstrual blood was a mystery as was amount and length of the period, and they were confused about body orifices. Hormonal influences were even less well understood, and many were not clear about when ovulation occurs (Koff & Rierdan, 1995).

The girls had, however, learned negative cultural stereptypes about menstruation and its symptoms such as cramps, backaches, bloating, and irritability. These are the messages that advertising for menstrual prod-

ucts reinforces. The findings of this study are congruent with a number of others including those of girls much older than 11 (Koff & Rierdan, 1995). A study of Finnish girls found their most frequent questions had to do with what is normal in menstruation and the menstrual cycle (Oinas, 1998). Other studies find that girls had strongly internalized cultural messages of menstruation as smelly and dirty and a source of shame, and that it must be concealed, especially from males (Lee & Sasser-Coen, 1996). Such beliefs are well entrenched in the culture and further reinforced in advertising for menstrual products. Physical discomforts such as cramps, backache, bloating, and breast tenderness are heavily emphasized in ads for products to relieve "symptoms." Psychological distress is fostered by recurrent advertising themes stressing protection, secrecy, and security to alleviate anxiety about odor, staining, and soiling and to achieve "peace of mind" (Koff & Rierdan, 1995).

Equally as important as knowledge of the physiological changes involved is the transformation to cultural norms of femininity, which girls are expected to make at menarche. These norms involve restrictions on previous activities and confusing messages about being sexually attractive but at the same time managing their own sexual feelings as well as those of boys. Such conflicting messages must be dealt with in educational programs (Lee & Sasser-Coen, 1996).

In order to better understand these attitudes, Morse and others (Morse, Kieren, & Bottorff, 1993; Morse & Kieren, 1993) have developed the Adolescent Menstrual Attitude Questionnaire with versions for pre-and postmenarcheal girls. The scales may be found in Tables 3.1 and 3.2. There are 47 parallel and 11 unique items on each questionnaire. Work on content validity has been done and six subscales identified, closely replicating the dimensions found on a qualitative study and thus supporting construct validity of the instruments. Items for the six subscales are: Positive feelings (21, 47, 32, 26, 45, 2, 24, 43, 28, 4, 15, 55 for premenarcheal; 47, 32, 45, 2, 28, 26, 43, 24, 21, 4, 52 for postmenarcheal); Negative feelings (10, 33, 8, 1, 41, 27, 5, 7, 42, 11, 48, 23, 5, 7, 18, 6, 52, 44 for premenarcheal; 33, 11, 40, 44, 11, 23, 18, 6, 10, 42, 41, 7, 49, 5, 54, 8, 57, 39 for postmenarcheal); Menstrual symptoms (30, 20, 34, 31, 14 for premenarcheal; 30, 34, 20, 31, 14, 56. 51, 50, 48 for postmenarcheal); Openess (22, 9, 16, 38, 39, 3 for premenarcheal; 9, 22, 16, 3, 38 for postmenarcheal); Acceptance of menarche (58, 37, 51, 13, 36, 19, 49, 40 for premenarcheal; 19, 13, 36, 15, 55, 27, 37 for postmenarcheal); Living with menstruation (25, 53, 35, 12, 56, 29, 17, 54, 50, 46 for premenarcheal; 58, 25, 17, 12, 46, 35, 53, 29 for postmenarcheal).

Items are scored 1 for strongly disagree and 5 for strongly agree except for the reverse-scored items as noted, with a total score of 58–

TABLE 3.1   Adolescent Menstrual Attitude Questionnaire, Premenarcheal Form

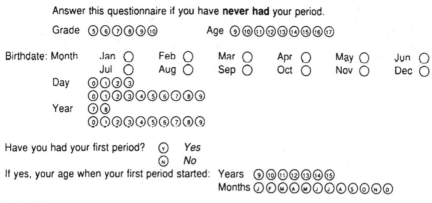

Answer this questionnaire if you have **never had** your period.

Grade ⑤⑥⑦⑧⑨⑩   Age ⑨⑩⑪⑫⑬⑭⑮⑯⑰

Birthdate: Month   Jan ○   Feb ○   Mar ○   Apr ○   May ○   Jun ○
                   Jul ○   Aug ○   Sep ○   Oct ○   Nov ○   Dec ○
          Day   ⓪①②③
                ⓪①②③④⑤⑥⑦⑧⑨
          Year ⑦⑧
                ⓪①②③④⑤⑥⑦⑧⑨

Have you had your first period?   ⓥ   *Yes*
                                  ⓝ   *No*
If yes, your age when your first period started: Years   ⑨⑩⑪⑫⑬⑭⑮
                                                   Months ⓙⒻⓜⒶⓜⒿⒿⒶⓈⓄⓃⒹ

Instructions

Next is a questionnaire concerning how girls feel about menstruation, *which is another word for your* period. *We will be asking you to indicate how much you agree, or disagree, with each statement, like this:*

1. I think boys should be told everything about girls periods.
   - ⓈⒹ   *means that you* strongly *disagree with the statement.*
   - Ⓓ   *means that you disagree with the statement, but you do not strongly disagree.*
   - Ⓝ   *means that you don't care, are not sure, or do not know.*
   - Ⓐ   *means that you agree with the statement.*
   - ⓈⒶ   *means that you* strongly *agree with the statement.*

Now, think about the statement, and fill in the circle next to the statement that is your own opinion. *There are no right or wrong answers. We are one interested in what* you think. *You do not have to answer any question that you do not want to. If you decide not to answer any questions at all, that's fine too, but we ask you to go to the other activity room.*

Please do not *put your name on this form. These answers ate your own personal opinions, and we consider your feelings private.*

1. When I have my period, I will be scared that the boys will find out.   ⓈⒹⒹⓃⒶⓈⒶ
2. It will make me feel very happy to know that I am finally menstruating.   ⓈⒹⒹⓃⒶⓈⒶ
3. I will not tell anyone when my period starts.   ⓈⒹⒹⓃⒶⓈⒶ
4. I was happy when I found out about menstruation.   ⓈⒹⒹⓃⒶⓈⒶ
5. I worry that one day I might not notice that I'm bleeding.   ⓈⒹⒹⓃⒶⓈⒶ

6. Most girls are bothered by buying pads or tampons at school or at a store.   ⓈⒹⒹⓃⒶⓈⒶ
7. I think I will feel uncomfortable when I have my period.   ⓈⒹⒹⓃⒶⓈⒶ
8. I am scared stiff at the thought of my period starting.   ⓈⒹⒹⓃⒶⓈⒶ
9. I often talk about periods with my friends.   ⓈⒹⒹⓃⒶⓈⒶ
10. I worry a lot about my periods starting.   ⓈⒹⒹⓃⒶⓈⒶ

11. Girls do not like to be seen putting pads in the garbage.   ⓈⒹⒹⓃⒶⓈⒶ
12. It is normal for girls to menstruate.   ⓈⒹⒹⓃⒶⓈⒶ
13. I will not feel any different than usual when I menstruate.   ⓈⒹⒹⓃⒶⓈⒶ
14. Girls who say they feel sick when they have their periods are just making excuses.   ⓈⒹⒹⓃⒶⓈⒶ
15. I we feel okay when I get my period.   ⓈⒹⒹⓃⒶⓈⒶ

(continued)

TABLE 3.1   (Continued)

O   SD = Strongly Disagree   D = Disagree   N = Nor Sure   A = Agree   SA = Strongly Agree

16. When I talk with my friends about periods I feel uncomfortable about it.   (SD) (D) (N) (A) (SA)
17. When girls have their period, they should be allowed to stay home.   (SD) (D) (N) (A) (SA)
18. Girls worry a lot that blood will leak through their clothes.   (SD) (D) (N) (A) (SA)
19. I will get used to periods very quickly.   (SD) (D) (N) (A) (SA)
20. Menstruating girls are grumpy and tense.   (SD) (D) (N) (A) (SA)

21. I look forward to getting my first period.   (SD) (D) (N) (A) (SA)
22. I like to talk about periods with my friends.   (SD) (D) (N) (A) (SA)
23. It's embarrassing to ask questions about periods.   (SD) (D) (N) (A) (SA)
24. When I get my period I will feel good.   (SD) (D) (N) (A) (SA)
25. Girls with periods should avoid exercise.   (SD) (D) (N) (A) (SA)

26. I will feel excited when I get my period.   (SD) (D) (N) (A) (SA)
27. I feel scared because I don't know what will happen when I get my period.   (SD) (D) (N) (A) (SA)
28. I will feel very grown up when I have my period.   (SD) (D) (N) (A) (SA)
29. When girls have their periods they should not shampoo their hair.   (SD) (D) (N) (A) (SA)
30. Girls are often grouchy when they have their periods.   (SD) (D) (N) (A) (SA)

31. When I get my period I expect I will feel sick.   (SD) (D) (N) (A) (SA)
32. I feel pleased when i think of starting my period.   (SD) (D) (N) (A) (SA)
33. When I start having my period, I am terrified that people will find out.   (SD) (D) (N) (A) (SA)
34. I expect to feel moody when I get my period.   (SD) (D) (N) (A) (SA)
35. Girls who get cramps with their period should worry something is wrong with them.   (SD) (D) (N) (A) (SA)

36. Coping with periods is easy.   (SD) (D) (N) (A) (SA)
37. Most girls understand what is happening to their body when they get a period.   (SD) (D) (N) (A) (SA)
38. Girls feel uncomfortable studying about menstruation at school.   (SD) (D) (N) (A) (SA)
39. I feel it's OK to discuss periods with boys.   (SD) (D) (N) (A) (SA)
40. Girls do not mind buying pads.   (SD) (D) (N) (A) (SA)

41. When I get my period, I will worry that people will be able to tell.   (SD) (D) (N) (A) (SA)
42. Every time someone mentions "period" I get nervous.   (SD) (D) (N) (A) (SA)
43. I am glad I am growing mature enough to menstruate.   (SD) (D) (N) (A) (SA)
44. Most girls find it embarrassing to get a pad from a public washroom machine   (SD) (D) (N) (A) (SA)
45. I will feel special when I get my period.   (SD) (D) (N) (A) (SA)

46. It is OK to swim when you have your period.   (SD) (D) (N) (A) (SA)
47. I will feel proud when I get my period.   (SD) (D) (N) (A) (SA)
48. The thought of getting my period is hard to get used to.   (SD) (D) (N) (A) (SA)
49. I do not care if my period starts or not.   (SD) (D) (N) (A) (SA)
50. I think I will walk differently when I am menstruating.   (SD) (D) (N) (A) (SA)

51. Getting my period will be no big deal.   (SD) (D) (N) (A) (SA)
52. I think periods are very dirty.   (SD) (D) (N) (A) (SA)
53. Girls who have their periods should not take a bath.   (SD) (D) (N) (A) (SA)
54. When girls have their periods, they should shower more frequently.   (SD) (D) (N) (A) (SA)
55. Having a period is a big nuisance.   (SD) (D) (N) (A) (SA)

56. Girls avoid talking to anyone about their concerns regarding periods.   (SD) (D) (N) (A) (SA)
57. I will feel shocked when my period begins.   (SD) (D) (N) (A) (SA)
58. Most girls understand exactly what to do when they get their first period.   (SD) (D) (N) (A) (SA)

TABLE 3.1 (Continued)

| WRITE IN THIS BOX ONLY |
| Have you thought of anything you would like to ask us? |
| |
| |
| Thank you for your help with this research!! |

From Morse, Janice M., Kiernen, Dianne, & Bottorff, Joan. (1993). The Adolescent Menstrual Attitude Questionnaire: Part I. Scale Construction. *Health Care for Women International, 14*:39–69. Copyright © 1993 Taylor and Francis.

290. A high score is indicative of a "positive" attitude and a low score of a "negative" attitude. Total test reliability (Cronbach's alpha) was .91 for the premenarcheal scale and .90 for the postmenarcheal scale. This level is adequate for group-level comparisons as well as diagnostic use in clinical settings. Although girls' attitudes toward menstruation are diverse, they became more positive with age as did severity of symptoms. Norms for girls in grades 6–9 may be found in Morse and Kiernen (1993).

One of the most difficult limitations to teaching menstrual self-care is the limited knowledge about menstruation and health consequences of the menstrual cycle. The medical textbook image of the 28-day menstrual cycle is an idealized model of the hormonal changes that occur during an ovulatory cycle. The majority of women, however, neither consistently experience 28-day cycles nor ovulate on day 14. Few quantitative data are available to explain how cycle length or bleed duration varies from cycle to cycle for a woman over time or how these patterns change as women age (Harlow & Ephross, 1995).

After menarche and before menopause, menstrual periods are more frequently extremely long or extremely short. In 10–14-year-old girls and in women more than 50 years of age, about a third of cycles are anovulatory compared with 2%–7% in the intervening years. The subtle changes that occur between the ages of 20 and 40 are not well described. Some women experience short menstrual cycles, whereas others have long cycles. Some seem prone to amenorrhea, others not, yet little is known about genetic factors in menstrual function. Weight, physical activity, and psychological stress do affect menstrual function. Women's self-reports of amount of bleeding have been found to be inaccurate and

TABLE 3.2 Adolescent Menstrual Attitude Questionnaire, Postmenarcheal Form

Answer this questionnaire if you have **never had** your period.

Grade ⑤⑥⑦⑧⑨⑩   Age ⑨⑩⑪⑫⑬⑭⑮⑯⑰

Birthdate: Month   Jan ○   Feb ○   Mar ○   Apr ○   May ○   Jun ○
            Jul ○   Aug ○   Sep ○   Oct ○   Nov ○   Dec ○

Day   ⓪①②③
      ⓪①②③④⑤⑥⑦⑧⑨

Year   ⑦⑧
      ⓪①②③④⑤⑥⑦⑧⑨

Have you had your first period?   ⓨ   Yes
                          ⓝ   No

If yes, your age when your first period started: Years   ⑨⑩⑪⑫⑬⑭⑮
                                                Months   ⒿⒻⓂⒶⓂⒿⒿⒶⓈⓄⓃⒹ

Instructions

Next is a questionnaire concerning how girls feel about menstruation, *which is another word for your* period. *We will be asking you to indicate how much you agree, or disagree, with each statement, like this:*

1. I think boys should be told everything about girls periods.
    ⓢⒹ   *means that you* strongly *disagree with the statement.*
    ⓓ   *means that you disagree with the statement, but you do not strongly disagree.*
    ⓝ   *means that you don't care, are not sure, or do not know.*
    ⓐ   *means that you agree with the statement.*
    ⓢⒶ   *means that you* strongly *agree with the statement.*

Now, think about the statement, and fill in the circle next to the statement that is your own opinion. *There are no right or wrong answers. We are one interested in what you think. You do not have to answer any question that you do not want to. If you decide not to answer any questions at all, that's fine too, but we ask you to go to the other activity room.*

Please do not put your name on this form. These answers ate your own personal opinions, and we consider your feelings private.

1. When I am having my period, I am scared that the boys will find out.   ⓢⒹⓓⓝⓐⓢⒶ
2. It makes me feel very happy to know that I am menstruating.   ⓢⒹⓓⓝⓐⓢⒶ
3. I have not told anyone that my periods have started.   ⓢⒹⓓⓝⓐⓢⒶ
4. I was happy when I found out about menstruation.   ⓢⒹⓓⓝⓐⓢⒶ
5. I worry that one day I might not notice that I'm bleeding.   ⓢⒹⓓⓝⓐⓢⒶ

6. Most girls are bothered by buying pads or tampons at school or at a store.   ⓢⒹⓓⓝⓐⓢⒶ
7. Just the fact that I have my period makes me uncomfortable.   ⓢⒹⓓⓝⓐⓢⒶ
8. I was scared stiff when my first period started.   ⓢⒹⓓⓝⓐⓢⒶ
9. I often talk about periods with my friends.   ⓢⒹⓓⓝⓐⓢⒶ
10. I worry a lot about my periods starting unexpectedly.   ⓢⒹⓓⓝⓐⓢⒶ

11. Girls do not like to be seen putting pads in the garbage.   ⓢⒹⓓⓝⓐⓢⒶ
12. It is normal for girls to menstruate.   ⓢⒹⓓⓝⓐⓢⒶ
13. I do not feel any different than usual when I menstruate.   ⓢⒹⓓⓝⓐⓢⒶ
14. Girls who say they feel sick from their periods are just making excuses.   ⓢⒹⓓⓝⓐⓢⒶ
15. I feel okay when I get my period.   ⓢⒹⓓⓝⓐⓢⒶ

TABLE 3.2 (Continued)

O SD = Strongly Disagree D = Disagree N = Not Sure A = Agree SA = Strongly Agree

16. When I talk with my friends about periods I feel uncomfortable about it. (SD) (D) (N) (A) (SA)
17. When girls have their period, they should be allowed to stay home. (SD) (D) (N) (A) (SA)
18. Girls worry a lot that blood will leak through their clothes. (SD) (D) (N) (A) (SA)
19. I quickly got used to having my periods. (SD) (D) (N) (A) (SA)
20. Menstruating girls are grumpy and tense. (SD) (D) (N) (A) (SA)

21. I couldn't wait to get my first period. (SD) (D) (N) (A) (SA)
22. I like to talk about periods with my friends. (SD) (D) (N) (A) (SA)
23. It's embarrassing to ask questions about periods. (SD) (D) (N) (A) (SA)
24. When I have my period I feel good. (SD) (D) (N) (A) (SA)
25. Girls with periods should avoid exercise. (SD) (D) (N) (A) (SA)

26. I feel excited when I get my period. (SD) (D) (N) (A) (SA)
27. I feel scared because I don't know what is happening when I have my period. (SD) (D) (N) (A) (SA)
28. I feel very grown up when I have my period. (SD) (D) (N) (A) (SA)
29. When girls have their periods they should not Shampoo their hair. (SD) (D) (N) (A) (SA)
30. Girls are often grouchy when they have their periods. (SD) (D) (N) (A) (SA)

31. When I get my period I feel sick. (SD) (D) (N) (A) (SA)
32. I feel pleased when I think of having a period. (SD) (D) (N) (A) (SA)
33. I am terrified that people will find out when I have my period. (SD) (D) (N) (A) (SA)
34. Girls feel moody when they get their period. (SD) (D) (N) (A) (SA)
35. Girls who get cramps with their period should worry something is wrong with them. (SD) (D) (N) (A) (SA)

36. Coping with periods is easy. (SD) (D) (N) (A) (SA)
37. Most girls understand what is happening to their body when they get a period. (SD) (D) (N) (A) (SA)
38. Girls feel uncomfortable studying about menstruation at school. (SD) (D) (N) (A) (SA)
39. I feel it's OK to discuss periods with boys. (SD) (D) (N) (A) (SA)
40. Girls do not mind buying pads. (SD) (D) (N) (A) (SA)

41. I feel people can tell when I have my period. (SD) (D) (N) (A) (SA)
42. Every time someone mentions "period" I get nervous. (SD) (D) (N) (A) (SA)
43. I am glad I have grown mature enough to menstruate. (SD) (D) (N) (A) (SA)
44. Most girls find getting a pad from a public washroom machine very embarrassing. (SD) (D) (N) (A) (SA)
45. I feel special when I have my period. (SD) (D) (N) (A) (SA)

46. It is OK to swim when you have your period. (SD) (D) (N) (A) (SA)
47. I feel proud when I have my period. (SD) (D) (N) (A) (SA)
48. Cramps during my period are very painful. (SD) (D) (N) (A) (SA)
49. When you have your period it is important to act cool, so no one will know. (SD) (D) (N) (A) (SA)
50. Girls get severe backaches with their periods. (SD) (D) (N) (A) (SA)

51. When girls get their periods they often feel like throwing up. (SD) (D) (N) (A) (SA)
52. When I began having my period, I changed into a woman. (SD) (D) (N) (A) (SA)
53. It's OK to miss school if you have cramps with your period. (SD) (D) (N) (A) (SA)
54. I feel ugly and gross when I have my period. (SD) (D) (N) (A) (SA)
55. When I am menstruating I feel the same. (SD) (D) (N) (A) (SA)

(continued)

TABLE 3.2 (Continued)

56. Girls cry more easily when they have their period. ⓈⒹⓄⓃⒶⓈⒶ
57. Girls dislike touching themselves to change their pads or tampons. ⓈⒹⓄⓃⒶⓈⒶ
58. When girls get their periods they should be excused from gym. ⓈⒹⓄⓃⒶⓈⒶ

> WRITE IN THIS BOX ONLY
> Have you thought of anything you would like to ask us?
>
>
>
>
> Thank you for your help with this research!!

From Morse, Janice M., Kiernen, Dianne, & Bottorff, Joan. (1993). The Adolescent Menstrual Attitude Questionnaire: Part I. Scale Construction. *Health Care for Women International, 14*:39–69. Copyright © 1993 Taylor and Francis.

therefore insufficient for clinical diagnosis of pathological conditions such as menorrhagia (Harlow & Ephross, 1995).

Considerable morbidity is directly attributable to menstrual disturbances. Dysmenorrhea involves abdominal pain, cramping, or backache associated with menstrual bleeding. It is experienced by 30%–60% of women of reproductive age and about 70% of young adult women, although it is severe enough to interfere with daily activity in only 7%–15%. Some changes in physiologic function during the menstrual cycle are understood, some not. Insulin sensitivity decreases during the luteal phase of the cycle, at least for a subset of patients. Little is understood about variation in immune competence across the cycle (Harlow & Ephross, 1995).

It is important to understand limitations of knowledge that thwart meeting the kind of educational objectives that would be useful to women in menstrual self-care. Population data on menstrual-cycle length and blood loss lack the detail on within-woman variability necessary to enable women and clinicians to anticipate specific bleeding changes that are likely to occur at different life stages, to differentiate potentially pathologic alterations from short-term aberrations, and to identify bleeding patterns that may be risk factors for the development of chronic disease. The absence of data that characterize bleeding changes as women approach and pass through the menopause is of particular concern given the frequency of physician visits for abnormal bleeding and the prevalence of hysterectomies after age 35 years. The fact that women have no comparative information on how much bleeding constitutes "too much" suggests that there is still a need for the development of objective criteria by which women can self-assess their daily blood loss, and more education is needed to inform women of what constitutes menstrual dysfunction. In addition, little is known about the natural variability in menstrual cycles across the reproductive life course in ethnically and economically diverse populations (Harlow & Ephross, 1995).

REPRODUCTION

Patient education should increase women's confidence in their ability to exercise control over disease and pregnancy. Feminists believe that this goal runs counter to the long-standing sexist assumption that women's role is to serve others (Purdy, 1996).

The goal is also thwarted by implicit policies (never formally adopted) that shape health benefits in a way that encourages births among working-and middle-class women and discourages births among the poor. Though poor women on Medicaid have mandated coverage of contraceptives, working- and middle-class women do not. Though the latter have mandated coverage of infertility in some jurisdictions, the few infertility benefits that were available to Medicaid recipients have not been repealed. Several states now mandate private insurers to cover infertility, but no state requires them to cover contraceptives. This flies in the face of the position that all women, regardless of social or economic class, should have the right and the means to control their reproductivity; such a goal requires access to a full range of reproductive benefits (King & Meyer, 1997).

Issues of pregnancy and birth are addressed in chapter 4, and the impact of sexually transmitted diseases on reproductive health is addressed in chapter 5. Approximately 60% of U. S. women of reproductive age use contraception but fewer than half are satisfied with the available methods (Wentz, 1994). Yet, contraceptive education is not well addressed in the literature and, as with other topics, much of it appears to be delivered by means of literature accompanying contraceptive drugs and devices.

Patient education plays an important role in assuring informed consent to and lack of regret after more permanent forms of contraception. A study of women who had undergone tubal sterilization found that the information received about the ligation itself and the number of contraceptive methods known to the woman at the time were significantly associated with regret. In this population of Brazilian women, poor counseling and limited access to reversible contraceptive methods resulted in an unacceptably high rate of request for reversal of sterilization. Women who declared that they had not been informed of the irreversibility of the procedure had an almost four times higher risk of requesting reversal of tubal ligation. Those who were not informed that they could change their minds at any time before surgery, about how the surgical procedure would be performed, or of the possibility of failure, also had a significantly increased risk of requestiong reversal (Hardy, Bahamondes, Osis, Losta, & Faundes, 1996).

According to internationally accepted guidelines, before being sterilized, women should receive complete information about the procedure and its possible consequences and complications. It is also recommended that women be informed about other available alternatives. The importance of adherence to these norms is strongly supported by the data from Hardy et al. (1996).

MENOPAUSE

Menopause is defined as the absence of menstrual periods for a year, which can be identified only retrospectively. Usually, menstrual cycles become shorter, then longer, and increasingly more variable before ceasing altogether (Mansfield & Voda, 1997).

Strong criticisms of the medicalization of menopause point out how aging that affects the reproductive capacities of men has been deftly passed over. Viewing menopause as subject to medical management, as being a transition that is costly to society because of disability from osteoporosis, and dismissal of the subjective experience and associated changes in human relationships are also criticized (Lock, 1993). Others (Mansfield & Voda, 1997) charge that the normal menopausal transition is poorly understood because data are based on clinical samples of White middle-class women and not on healthy women, which means that it is difficult for women and for health care providers who advise them to interpret symptoms. The specific changes vary from woman to woman. One of the most alarming symptoms for women is the onset of very heavy bleeding that usually stains right through clothing. They equate this symptom with a disease, usually cancer. Women can cope successfully with a wide variety of conditions once they know they are within normal range.

Popular images and stereotypes of women in the menopausal age range are overwhelmingly negative, suggesting that the transition is stressful, disruptive, depressive, and a time of decline when it can be experienced as a time of liberation and creativity. The biomedical view of menopause is as a deficiency disease with a long list of negative symptoms related exclusively to physiology. This view suggests that women are weaker and sicker than the normal male ideal. It pathologizes women's natural aging processes. Alternate views suggest that menopause is not particularly problematic for most women and that the establishment of medical authority over it disempowers women. Every woman over 50 becomes a patient. These critics see the currently dominant view of menopause as a political phenomenom disguised as medical science, which can be harmful to women (Rostosky & Travis, 1996).

Surveys of women at midlife describe a perceived unresponsiveness of the health care system to their need for information about the menopausal transition. Because most educational materials are underwritten by pharmaceutical companies, it is not easy for women to find information on alternative, nonhormonal therapies for menopausal ailments; those who have reservations about hormone replacement therapy (HRT) may feel they have no choices (Mansfield & Voda, 1997).

Figure 3.1 reproduces an information booklet on management of menopausal symptoms. Nurses are often frustrated by the lack of literature of this sort. Appropriate management of menopausal symptoms is becoming more of an issue as more and more conflicting and often confusing studies on the role of HRT are published in the lay press. Women with a history of breast cancer, those at increased risk for breast cancer, or others with cancer who have received menopause-inducing treatments may have additional concerns about managing these symptoms (Mayer & Linscott, 1995).

Postmenopausal Osteoporosis

The number of postmenopausal women in the United States will approach 60 million in the next decade. Osteoporosis affects half of women over age 45, 90% of women over 75, and is a common cause of significant morbidity and disability. Women are about six times more likely to be affected than are men. Postmenopausal osteoporosis is a

FIGURE 3.1   **Management of menopausal symptoms.**

INTRODUCTION

This figure addresses common questions raised about how to handle the symptoms of menopause. It is not meant to give specific information for an individual woman. It's meant to raise questions and provide resources to find answers to those questions. Specific information should be obtained from the woman's health care professional.

What Changes Occur
DURING MENOPAUSE?

Menopause is the end of menstruation when a woman stops having menstrual periods. Menopause often refers to the time when these changes occur and also may be referred to as change of life, the climacteric, or perimenopause. This generally occurs with women in their early 50s but may occur anytime between the ages of 40 and 60. Menopause occurs because a woman's body no longer naturally makes enough of the hormones needed to produce her period. The process of menopause may be gradual or abrupt. Some women with cancer may experience their change of life prematurely because of their treatment or cancer.

Each woman may react differently to menopause. A number of changes can occur. Not all women will experience the same thing or in the same way. Some of these changes include

- Hot flashes and sweats
- Sleep disturbances
- Vaginal dryness
- Urinary tract changes
- Skin changes
- Mood changes
- Sex drive changes.

Other important changes also occur that are not immediately noticed. Bones begin to lose calcium and may weaken. (This is known as osteoporosis.) The heart and blood vessels may weaken, and heart disease may develop.

A woman's quality of life (QOL) can be affected by the number, length, and degree of these-symptoms. Many women manage this change of life with little difficulty. Some women with more concerns or symptoms may worry about how to manage them.

Women with breast cancer, those who are at increased risk for breast cancer, or others with cancer who have received menopause-causing treatments also may have special concerns.

What Can I Do
ABOUT MENOPAUSE?

Many women want to know what they pan do to adapt to these changes and promote their health during menopause. Women should make sure that they

- Have enough calcium in their diet (between 1000–1500 mg/day [this dose should not be exceeded]).
- Eat foods that are low in fat and high in fiber.
- Exercise regularly (at least 30 minutes, three times/week).

FIGURE 3.1 **(Continued)**

What Is Hormonal
REPLACEMENT THERAPY?

Many women also have questions about whether or not they should receive hormone replacement therapy (HRT). Many studies have focused on HRT, but the results often are conflicting or confusing. It is difficult to know what the right thing to do is.

HRT may be recommended for short- or long-term use. Short-term use can last up to five years and is for the relief of menopause symptoms such as hot flashes or vaginal dryness. Long-term use lasts 10 or more years and may reduce the risk of heart disease and bone loss.

There are different types and methods of HRT. For example, it can be administered in the form of pills, a skin patch, or a cream. It can be given as estrogen alone or in combinations with progesterone.

Use of long-term HRT may affect a woman's length, as well as quality, of life. Although HRT frequently is recommended in the general population, its use slightly increases the risk of breast cancer.

HRT use is more controversial in women with a history or greater risk of breast cancer. The risk of breast cancer does increase for some of these women. Conventional medical advice generally has been to avoid the use of HRT, but this advice is being reconsidered. There are no clear answers about what any one woman should do.

Some side effects of HRT include irregular bleeding, bloating, and breast tenderness. Endometrial cancers are experienced by more women when estrogen is used alone, if they have not had a hysterectomy. A combination of hormones (estrogen and progesterone) is recommended to reduce this risk.

Risks and benefits for an individual woman must be discussed prior to making an informed decision about HRT use. Other nonhormonal medications also can be used in managing hot flashes, but they may be less effective. You may want to discuss this, and other options, with your healthcare provider.

Questions and Concerns
to Discuss With Your
HEALTHCARE PROVIDER*

- Should I take hormones? If so, why?
- If breast cancer has occurred in my family, should I take hormones?
- If I have had breast cancer, should I take hormones?
- How will hormones improve my risk for heart disease or osteoporosis? How will hormones improve my menopausal symptoms?
- What side effects might I expect?
- At what age should I begin taking hormones?
- How long should I take hormones?
- What should I do if I start taking hormones?

*Adapted from Hormone replacement therapy and heart disease: The PEPI Trial. *NIH Publication 95–3277 (August 1995).*

FIGURE 3.1   **(Continued)**

TABLE 1. AVERAGE WOMAN'S CHANCES OF DEVELOPING AND DYING FROM SELECTED CONDITIONS

Risk Factor	Lifetime Probability of Development (and Death)	Median Age at Development
Coronary heart disease	46% (31%)	74
Stroke	20% (8%)	83
Osteoporotic hip fracture	15% (2%)	79
Breast cancer (increased risk)	19% –	–
Breast cancer (average ask)	10% (3%)	69
Endometrial cancer[a]	3% (.3%)	68

[a]Calculated for a woman with a uterus (chances are zero if the woman has had a hysterectomy)

Note. Based on information from Grady et al. (1992).

What Are Some Other Ways to Manage MENOPAUSAL SYMPTOMS?

A variety of other remedies have been used to help manage symptoms during menopause. Most of these remedies have not been scientifically studied but have been helpful for some women. These include

- Dressing in layers and natural fibers (e.g., cotton)
- Regular exercise
- Stress reduction (e.g., relaxation techniques, yoga)
- Nutrition changes (e.g., reducing or avoiding caffeine and alcohol)
- Homeopathy
- Herbalism
- Traditional Chinese medicines
- Vitamin and mineral supplements
- Talking with other women.

Before a woman decides what she wants to do, she may want to read some of the references provided at the end of this booklet for specific ideas as well as discuss her situation with her doctor or nurse. Referrals to registered dieticians are also available.

Hormonal Therapy AND MENOPAUSAL DATA

Table 1 identifies lifetime probability of getting and dying from one of the listed conditions. Table 2 may be helpful in considering the possible benefits and risks of taking hormones. The use of this table may help some women in asking questions or making decisions.

FIGURE 3.1 (Continued)

Life expectancy for a 50–year-old white woman without known risk factors is 82.8 years. The net change in life expectancy with estrogen or estrogen plus progesterone ranges from –0.5 to +2.2 years based on risk factors and type of hormonal replacement. The data in these two tables reflect the risks and benefits of an average 50–year-old white woman. For example, this woman has a 46% chance of developing coronary heart disease during her lifetime. The average age at the time of developing heart disease is 74 years. She has a 31% chance of dying from heart disease. If she takes estrogen, the risk of developing heart disease is reduced from 46% to 34% with estrogen alone or from 46% to 39% if she uses estrogen and progesterone.

TABLE 2. BENEFITS AND RISKS OF HORMONE REPLACEMENT THERAPY (HRT)

Risk Factor	Lifetime Probability With HRT: Estrogen	Lifetime Probability With HRT: Estrogen and Progesterone
Coronary heart disease	34%	39%
Stroke	20%	19%
Osteoporotic hip fracture	13%	12%
Breast cancer (increased risk)	24%	35%
Breast cancer (average risk)	13%	20%
Endometrial cancer[a]	20%	3%

[a]Calculated for a woman with a uterus (Chances are zero if the woman has had a hysterectomy.)

Note. Based on information from Grady et al. (1992).

This booklet was developed by Deborah K. Mayer, RN, MSN, AOCN, FAAN, and Elizabeth Linscott, RN, and produced by the Princess Margaret Hospital (PMH) Patient Education Committee. It is reprinted with permission from PMH.

disorder characterized by decreased bone mass and increased susceptibility to fracture. It causes more than 1.5 million fractures of the hip, vertebrae, wrists, and other bones per year. Of the 250,000 hip fractures per year, 80% are in women, and mortality in the first year after a hip fracture is increased by more than 20% (Wentz, 1994).

Many reports suggest that most women are not well informed about menopause and that most get their information from the media. This information is probably insufficiently detailed and not adapted for individual patients. The Osteoporosis Health Belief, Self-Efficacy and Knowledge tests, developed by Kim, Horan, Gendler, and Patel (1991) are useful for assessment before education and evaluation afterward. These tests and a critique of them may be found in Redman (1998).

Because there is no cure for osteoporosis, prevention efforts are essential. Consuming at least 1,000 milligrams of calcium daily and engaging in 3 to 4 hours of weight-bearing exercise per week are recommended to reduce the risk of developing osteoporosis. Data from a variety of sources suggest that many women do not practice these behaviors. A stage model (precaution-adoption process model) conceptualizes behavior change as a process that evolves over time and has been studied for adoption of calcium and exercise behaviors to prevent osteoporosis (Blalock et al., 1996).

This model suggests that at any point in time a person will be in one of seven stages with respect to adoption of each precaution:

Stage 1: Unaware of health problem and the recommended precaution.
Stage 2: Aware of health problem and precaution but has never thought seriously about adopting the precaution.
Stage 3: Considered adopting the precaution but decided against it.
Stage 4: Trying to decide whether to adopt the precaution.
Stage 5: Decided to adopt the precaution.
Stage 6: Acted on that decision.
Stage 7: Maintained the precaution for a substantial period of time.

A stages-of-change model allows more precise interventions tailored to the stage of change for an individual and a particular behavior. Blalock et al. (1996) used the precaution-adoption process model on the behaviors of calcium consumption and weight-bearing exercise. They found that many more women were in the currently engaged stage for exercise than for calcium.

The decision to begin HRT as a means to prevent osteoporosis is a large one. Many women are dissatisfied with the information they are receiving from their physicians about menopause in general as well as about HRT. They report that they rely on lay media reports, which have largely ignored the benefits of HRT, including its potential to prevent cardiovascular disease. A large percentage of women who discontinue HRT do so because they fear cancer (Witt & Lousberg, 1997). Women who were aware that they had lower than average bone mineral density were more likely to continue HRT (Rozenberg, Vasques, Vandromme, & Kroll, 1998).

Only 15%–25% of those eligible for HRT make use of it, and many stay on it for only a brief time. Only 15% of those who take it at all stay on the regimen for 10 years or more (Silverman, Greenwald, Klein, & Drinkwater, 1997). It is also not easy for women to find information on alternative, nonhormonal therapies for postmenopausal ailments because most educational materials are underwritten by pharmaceutical companies whose interest is in promoting hormones (Mansfield & Voda, 1997).

Available evidence shows some differences in the menopause experience of White and African American women. In one study, White women were more than twice as likely to report that their physicians had inquired about menopausal symptoms, and significantly more often to have HRT recommended. Most studies of postmenopausal osteoporosis have included White women. Regardless of educational level, African American women are 60% less likely to have ever taken HRT than are White women (Rozenberg et al., 1998). Pham, Grisso, and Freeman (1997) report that African American women viewed menopause more positively than did White women, despite reporting symptoms similar in degree and frequency. A broader review of this literature describes conflicting findings about whether there are differences. There is evidence of less bone loss and higher breast cancer risks for African Americans who have experienced natural menopause. In general, ethnic groups have been underrepresented in research about menopause as have poor and working-class women. This is unfortunate because only when a wide range of experiences of the menopausal transition for healthy women are identified will it be possible for aging women and their providers to make accurate assessments of their individual patterns of change (Rousseau & McCool, 1997).

The decision about whether to go on HRT is value laden and involves trade-offs among possible risks of heart disease, osteoporosis, cancer, and menopausal symptoms. Because so many of these factors are individualized, general educational materials are limited in helping women judge their individualized risks and benefits. Decision aids differ from usual patient-education materials by focusing on alternatives, benefits, and risks tailored to a woman's clinical risk profile for heart disease, osteoporosis, and breast cancer; using explicit probabilities to describe the likelihood of benefits and risks; including values clarification to encourage evaluation of the personal importance of the risks and benefits; and emphasizing choice and shared decision making. The goal is to improve the quality of decision making by addressing modifiable suboptimal determinants of decisions: inadequate knowledge, unrealistic ex-

TABLE 3.3   Decision Support Framework

Assess client & practitioner determinants of decisions	Provide decision support Prepare practitioner & client for DM; structure follow-up interaction	Evaluate quality of decision and decision-making process	Evaluate client outcomes of decision
Sociodemographic & Clinical Characteristics	Tailor to participants' characteristics	Satisfaction with decision support & decision-making process	Improved health-related quality of life
Perception of the Decision knowledge expectations values decisional conflict	Provide access to information Clarify/modify expectations Clarify values Tailor support to factors contributing to decisional conflict	Improved knowledge Realistic expectations Improved clarity of values & value congruence with decision Reduced decisional conflict Reduced decision delay Satisfaction with decision	Reduced distress from consequences Reduced regret Appropriate persistence with decision
Perception of Important Others norms pressure support decision participation roles Resources to Make & Implement Decision	Clarify/modify perceived norms Clarify pressure; Facilitate Self-help skills handling pressure Facilitate access to support Tailor support to decision participation preferences	Realistic perception of norms and pressure Satisfaction with decision support	Appropriate persistence with decision
Personal resources experience self-efficacy skills motivation other resources	Enhance self-help skills preparing for, making, and implementing decisions and coping with consequences	Improved self-efficacy Improved decision making skills Decision implementation	Reduced distress from consequences Appropriate persistence with decision
External resources	Facilitate access to resources	Improved knowledge of resources	Appropriate end efficient use of resources Satisfaction with care

Reprinted from *Patient Education & Counseling, 33,* O'Connor, A. M., Tugwell, P., Wells, G. A., Elmslie, T., Jolly, E., Hollingworth, G., McPherson, R., Bunn, H., Graham, I., & Drake, E. (1998). A decision aid for women considering hormone therapy after menopause: Decision support framework and evaluation, pp. 267–279, with permission from Elsevier Science.

pectations, unclear values and norms, and inadequate support. A high-quality decision is defined as informed, consistent with personal values, acted on, and in which decision makers express satisfaction with the process and the decision. The Decision Support Framework may be found in Table 3.3 (O'Connor et al., 1998).

O'Connor et al. (1998) developed a self-administered HRT decision aid: a 40-minute audiotape that guided a woman through an illustrated booklet containing the elements listed previously, and a personal worksheet that included identification of personal lifetime benefits and risks of HRT, values clarification using a "weigh scale" and other elements. The "weigh scale" may be found in Figure 3.2. Women shaded a portion

Weigh scale profile of women who choose yes:

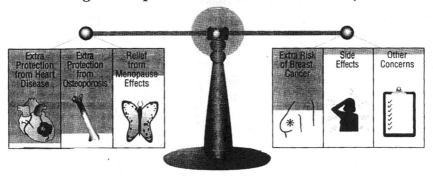

Weigh scale profile of women who choose no:

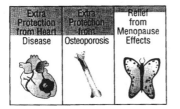
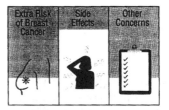

Weigh scale profile of women who are unsure:

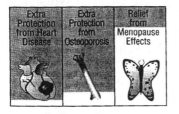
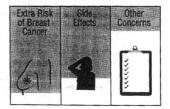

FIGURE 3.2   Weigh scale profile.

Reprinted from *Patient Education & Counseling, 33,* O'Connor, A. M., Tugwell, P., Wells, G. A., Elmslie, T., Jolly, E., Hollingworth, G., McPherson, R., Bunn, H., Graham, I., & Drake, E. A decision aid for women considering hormone therapy after menopause: Decision support framework and evaluation, pp. 267–279, with permission from Elsevier Science.

of each benefit and risk box to indicate how important it was to them (no shading indicating not at all important, completely shaded indicating extremely important). Most changes in preferences occurred in the initially uncertain group. Helping individuals to actively consider a decision in the context of their clinical risks and values provides the opportunity not only to improve the quality of the decision but also to increase self-efficacy and sense of mastery and control.

Rothert and others (1997) completed a randomized controlled trial comparing the performance of a decision support intervention to assist women to make and act on informed decisions in the area of menopause and HRT with written information only and guided discussion. At baseline, even this well-educated sample did not have adequate information on which to base a decision. All three interventions helped women to decrease decisional conflict, be satisfied with their decision, and feel self-efficacy to deal with the health care system. Although decision aids are in early stages of development, they show promise as a method by which to reach large numbers of menopausal women.

URINARY INCONTINENCE

Urinary incontinence (UI) is the involuntary loss of urine. It is much more common in women, affects as many as 8 million older women and is the tenth leading cause for hospitalization in the United States. Approximately half of nursing-home residents are incontinent. Approximately 20% of women ages 25–64 years experience UI, with symptoms frequently increasing during perimenopause and increasing with parity. It currently takes an average woman with urine leakage 1.6 years before discussing her condition with a physician, and 41% believe the problem is not severe enough to consult a health care provider (Sampselle et al., 1997).

Many women modify their lifestyles by wearing pads, avoiding travel, assuring easy access to bathrooms, modifying the type of clothes worn, and giving up exercise and intimacy. Because knowledge and skills for how to deal with UI are so difficult to obtain and yet the condition so debilitating, the Profiles of Women with Stress Incontinence Program targets health care providers and women. The Bladder Control help line is 1–800–526–2687 (Haller, 1997).

The most common type of UI is stress incontinence. A well-described set of tools including a screening questionnaire, voiding diary, bladder training program, and pelvic muscle instructions is available in Sampselle et al. (1997). Bladder training consists of asking patients to hold on for longer and longer before using the toilet and also toileting at regular intervals. It requires that the pelvic muscles are in good shape, patients are therefore taught to do exercises that give them confidence in bladder training (O'Brien, Austin, Sethi & O'Boyle, 1991). "How to Do Your Pelvic Floor Exercises" may be found in Table 3.4. To re-educate the correct muscle action, women must be able to squeeze, lift, hold, and relax the pelvic floor. Verbal and written instruction must be supplemented with performance feedback about how the muscle is contracting (Dolman, 1997).

In the Netherlands, Teleac, a broadcasting company for adult education, did training therapy for UI with 140,000 viewers per broadcast.

TABLE 3.4   How to Do Your Pelvic Floor Exercises

1. Sit comfortably with knees slightly apart. Without moving your tummy muscle or bottom, try to squeeze the muscle around the back passage. Pretend you are trying to stop wind from escaping!
2. Now try the same with the front part of the muscle. Again, without moving the tummy or bottom, squeeze and lift the muscle into the vagina. Moving this front part of the muscle is harder than that mentioned above and takes time to practice.
3. Once you can tighten and lift the muscles (lifting is as though you are taking the muscle up steps one at a time), pull as hard as you can and hold for as long as you can (e.g. 5 seconds), then relax. Repeat this 5–10 times with a good 'rest' between each contraction. Do the group of 5–10 exercises as many times a day without making your muscle ache.
4. Also try to squeeze your muscle quickly like a one-second 'flick,' then relax. Repeat this five times. Only do this once before your group of slow contractions.
5. These two actions of moving your muscle—i.e., slowly and then fast—will strengthen the pelvic floor muscle so that you will be able to do more repetitions and hold the squeeze longer. This will make the muscles strong and powerful.
6. To help you identify the correct muscles, you may wish to try placing two fingers into your vagina and then squeezing around the fingers with the pelvic floor muscles only. This could be tried when you are in the bath.
7. If in doubt about exercising properly, then do not hesitate to contact your healthcare provider who should be able to advise you.
8. Pelvic floor exercises are an important aspect of health promotion for all women.

From Dolman, Mary. Mostly female, pp. 68–106 in Getliffe, Kathryn, & Dolman, Mary (Eds.). (1997). *Promoting Continence: A Clinical and Research Resource*. London: Bailliere Tindall. Reprinted with permission W. B. Saunders Company Ltd.

Based on the view that medicalization of UI is unnecessary, the training package includes television and radio lessons and a textbook. Participants were given assignments such as keeping a record of their urinary loss and habits, and exercises to train the pelvic muscles. The television lessons covered the content in the book in visual form. Step-by-step guidance in improving the incontinence was provided. After the course, 51% of participants experienced improvement in their UI. Such an approach has the benefit of also reaching the social networks of those suffering from incontinence as well as health professionals (Niewijk & Weijts, 1997).

Few of the current management strategies (pelvic exercises, appliances, drugs, and surgery) have been the subject of well-designed randomized controlled trials (RCTs) in primary care, and few studies have reported long-term results. Thus, lack of evidence combined with poorly trained primary care physicians and nurses has meant that fewer than one in three patients is recognized and fewer still appropriately managed (O'Brien et al., 1991).

The role of a specialist nurse continence adviser was first developed in England and has grown extensively with 350 practicing in clinics and in community nursing by 1991. In addition to direct care, these advisers train other health professionals to ensure availability of knowledgeable incontinence care (Rhodes & Parker, 1995). In the UK, an RCT of the management of incontinence in primary care using a nurse trained in assessment and management techniques found a cure rate of 68% or improvement after 12 weeks in the intervention group, compared with 5% in the control group. The intervention consisted of four sessions of pelvic floor exercises and bladder retraining, depending on the dominant symptoms. Women were encouraged to continue the management plan at home. Women with stress incontinence were more likely to benefit than were those with urge incontinence or a combination of the two. Improvement was strongly associated with session attendance (O'Brien & Long, 1991).

Patient-centered evaluation of outcomes of surgical treatment for stress incontinence showed that a year after surgery, 68% would recommend it to a friend with only 28% achieving continence. This is in contrast to textbook and surgeons' claims of up to 85% achieving continence. Seventeen percent reported no benefit from the operation. Postoperative complications were more common than previously thought with one in six women reporting difficulty urinating for up to 3 months after surgery and a high prevalence of inadequately controlled pain. This information is important for informed consent when considering surgery (Black, Griffiths, Pope, Bowling, & Abel, 1997).

At least three health-related quality-of-life (HRQOL) instruments specific to UI are available. Shumaker, Wyman, Uebersax, McClish, and

Fantl (1994) describe the Urogenital Distress Inventory (UDI) and the Incontinence Impact Questionnaire (IIQ). Either or both could be used along with other instruments to evaluate treatment programs which include patient education. These measures provide data on the more traditional view of HRQOL by assessing the impact of UI on various activities, roles, and emotional states as well as data on the less traditional but critical issue of the degree to which symptoms associated with UI are troubling to women. Data on the reliability, validity, and sensitivity to change of these measures demonstrate that for the most part they are psychometrically strong. Content validity was supported by interviews with affected women and with health providers experienced in the assessment and treatment of UI. Scores on both the UDI and IIQ correlated strongly with measures of incontinence. Scoring directions may be found in the original sources.

Wagner, Patrick, Bavendam, Martin, and Buesching (1996) report on the Incontinence Quality of Life (I-QOL) measure. It too was developed from interviews of individuals with UI, with women comprising two thirds of the sample. Cronbach's alpha, a measure of internal consistency, was .95. Validity checks were done with other psychological instruments but not with clinically objective measures of UI severity, such as the perineal pad test. Sample items include: I worry about wetting myself; I worry about coughing or sneezing because of my incontinence; my incontinence makes me feel helpless.

SUMMARY

What is startling about the health concerns reviewed in this chapter is the lack of accessible knowledge available to women, and the attitudes of shame and concealment that accompany them. Well-designed, easily available education programs on these topics could do so much to empower women and contribute to their well-being.

REFERENCES

Black, N., Griffiths, J., Pope, C., Bowling, A., & Abel, P. (1997). Impact of surgery for stress incontinence on morbidity: Cohort study. *British Medical Journal, 315,* 1493–1498.

Blalock, S. J., DeVellis, R. F., Giorgino, K. B., DeVellis, B. M., Gold, D. T., Dooley, M. A., Anderson, J. J. B., & Smith, S. L. (1996). Osteoporosis prevention in premenopausal women: Using a stage model approach to examine the predictors of behavior. *Health Psychology, 15,* 84–93.

Dolman, M. (1997). Mostly female. In K. Getliffe & M. Dolman (Eds.), *Promoting continence; a clinical and research resource.* London: Balliere Tindall.

Grady, D., Rubin, S., Petitti, D., Fox, C., Black, D., Ettinger, B., Einster, V., & Cummings, S. (1992). Hormone therapy to prevent disease and prolong life in postmenopausal women. *Annals of Internal Medicine, 117,* 1016–1037.

Haller, K. B. (1997). Coming out of the (water) closet. *Journal of Obstetric, Gynecological, and Neonatal Nursing, 26,* 370.

Hardy, E., Bahamondes, L., Osis, M. J., Costa, R. G., & Faundes, A. (1996). Risk factors for tubal sterilization regret, detectable before surgery. *Contraception, 54,* 159–162.

Harlow, S. D., & Ephross, S. A. (1995). Epidemiology of menstruation and its relevance to women's health. *Epidemiologic Reviews, 17,* 265–286.

Kim, K. K., Horan, M. L., Gendler, P., & Patel, M. K. (1991). Development and evaluation of the Osteoporosis Health Belief Scale. *Research in Nursing and Health, 14,* 115–163.

King, L., & Meyer, M. H. (1997). The politics of reproductive benefits. *Gender and Society, 11,* 8–30.

Koff, E., & Rierdan, J. (1995). Early adolescent girls' understanding of menstruation. *Women & Health 22(4),* 1–19.

Lee, J., & Sasser-Coen, J. (1996). *Blood stories.* New York: Routledge.

Lock, M. (1993). The politics of mid-life and menopause. In S. Lindenbaum & M. Lock (Eds.), *Knowledge, power & practice.* Berkeley, CA: University of California Press.

Mansfield, P. K., & Voda, A. M. (1997). Woman-centered information on menopause for health care providers: Findings from the midlife women's health survey. *Health Care for Women International, 18,* 55–72.

Mayer, D. K., & Linscott, E. (1995). Information for women: Management of menopausal symptoms. *Oncology Nursing Forum, 22,* 1567–1570.

Morse, J. M., Kieren, D., & Bottorff, J. L. (1993). The Adolescent Menstrual Attitude Questionnaire: Part I. Scale construction. *Health Care for Women International, 14,* 39–69.

Morse, J. M., & Kieren, D. (1993). The Adolescent Menstrual Attitude Questionnaire: Part II. Normative scores. *Health Care for Women International, 14,* 63–76.

Niewijk, A. H., & Weitjs, B. M. W. (1997). Effects of a multi-media course on urinary incontinence. *Patient Education & Counseling, 30,* 95–103.

O'Brien, J., Austin, M., Sethi, P., & O'Boyle, P. (1991). Urinary incontinence:

Prevalence, need for treatment, and effectiveness of intervention by nurse. *British Medical Journal, 303,* 1308–1312.

O'Brien, J., & Long, H. (1995). Urinary incontinence: Long term effectiveness of nursing intervention in primary care. *British Medical Journal, 311,* 1208.

O'Connor, A. M., Tugwell, P., Wells, G. A., Elmslie, T., Jolly, E., Hollingworth, G., McPherson, R., Bunn, H., Graham, I., & Drake, E. (1998). A decision aid for women considering hormone therapy after menopause: Decision support framework and evaluation. *Patient Education and Counseling, 33,* 267–279.

Oinas, E. (1998). Medicalisation by whom? Accounts of menstruation conveyed by young women and medical experts in medical advisory columns. *Sociology of Health & Illness, 20,* 52–70.

Pham, K., Grisso, J. A., & Freeman, E. W. (1997). Ovarian aging and hormone replacement therapy. *General Internal Medicine, 12,* 230–236.

Purdy, L. M. (1996). What can progress in reproductive technology mean for women? *Journal of Medicine & Philosophy, 21,* 499–514.

Redman, B. K. (1998). *Measurement tools in patient education.* New York: Springer Publishing Co.

Rhodes, P., & Parker, G. (1995). The role of the continence adviser in England & Wales. *International Journal of Nursing Studies, 32,* 423–433.

Rostosky, S. S., & Travis, C. B. (1996). Menopause research & the dominance of the biomedical model 1984–1994. *Psychology of Women Quarterly, 20,* 285–312.

Rothert, M. L., Holmes-Rouner, M., Rouner, D., Kroll, J., Breer, L., Talarczyk, G., Schmitt, N., Padonu, G., & Wills, C. (1997). An educational intervention as decision support for menopausal women. *Research in Nursing & Health, 20,* 377–387.

Rousseau, M. E., & McCool, W. F. (1997). The menopausal experience of African American women: Overview and suggestions for research. *Health Care for Women International, 18,* 233–250.

Rozenberg, S., Vasquez, J. B., Vandromme, J., & Kroll, M. (1998). Educating patients about the benefits and drawbacks of hormone replacement therapy. *Drugs & Aging, 13,* 33–41.

Sampselle, C. M., Burns, P. A., Dougherty, M. C., Newman, D. K., Thomas, K. K., & Wyman, J. F. (1997). Continence for women: Evidence-based practice. *Journal of Obstetric, Gynecological, and Neonatal Nursing, 26,* 375–385.

Shumaker, S. A., Wyman, J. F., Uebersax, J. S., McClish, D., & Fantl, J. A. (1994). Health-related quality of life measures for women with urinary incontinence: The Incontinence Impact Questionnaire & the Urogenital Distress Inventory. *Quality of Life Research, 3,* 291–306.

Silverman, S. L., Greenwald, M., Klein, R. A., & Drinkwater, B. L. (1997).

Effect of bone density information on decisions about hormone replacement therapy: A randomized trial. *Obstetrics & Gynecology, 89,* 321–325.

Wagner, T. H., Patrick, D. L., Bavendam, T. G., Martin, M. L., & Buesching, D. P. (1996). Quality of life of persons with urinary incontinence: Development of a new measure. *Urology, 47,* 67–72.

Wentz, A. C. (1994). Women's health issues. *Advances in Internal Medicine, 40,* 1–30.

Witt, D. M., & Lousberg, T. R. (1997). Controversies surrounding estrogen use in postmenopausal women. *Annals of Pharmacotherapy, 31,* 745–755.

CHAPTER FOUR

Motherhood As Learning

Motherhood offers and requires profound learning and exposes personal strengths and resourcefulness. Throughout history, these learning opportunities have been deeply embedded in cultures through experiences in attending births and participating in the rearing of babies and small children. With the medicalization of childbirth and childrearing and geographic dispersion of families, for middle- and upper-class women, preparation for these roles has been incorporated in the health system. The medical profession did not share its knowledge with the women for whom it cared, and antenatal education attempted to replace the factual information and emotional insights traditionally transmitted through the women's network. Those from lower socioeconomic classes retained more access to an informal educational network and less frequently participated in formal antenatal education (Nolan, 1997).

These education services and the entire system for dealing with women's reproductive functions have been heavily criticized. Prenatal education is seen as focused on helping women fit into the existing system of maternity services, to encourage cooperation with health professionals caring for them, and avoid challenging physicians. The system is believed to have denied women freedom and choice in childbirth and has been labelled conformist, patronizing, and disempowering. Its contribution to health of the mother and neonate are said to be unclear (Nolan, 1997).

It is charged that antenatal education has avoided topics such as stillbirth, handicapped and very sick babies, and women who have long-term sequelae including mental health problems from giving birth, as well as basic baby-care skills and skills in accessing support. There is a sense among some that antenatal education does not prepare for the reality of birth, the unrelenting demands of infant care, the level of fatigue, feelings of being unprepared, and the loss of personal time new motherhood brings (McVeigh, 1997) and is a form of indoctrination. It is charged that medical model programs have the negative side effect of persuading women that their bodies are not capable of giving birth with-

out technological assistance. Because pregnancy and childbirth education are essential components of prenatal care for all women, it is important
to determine whether such a message truly is being given (Zwelling, 1996).

Feminist scholars have contended that the medical management of
reproductive processes has focused on societal and family needs and not
on those of the women involved. Risk has been assigned to individuals
rather than to structural and social conditions. The regular use of episiotomy, drugs, intrapartum electronic fetal monitoring and other technologies has been legitimated. It is charged that routine high-risk management
for normal pregnancy is not necessarily effective and may be seen as a
means of social control. It brings about acquiescence to medical interventions and norms because not to do so would be defined as irrespon-
sible. This moral high ground has rarely been challenged because
physicians have sufficient political power to sustain it and have been
able to convince the public that it is misinformed and behind in medical
innovation. Medical science has proceeded largely undeterred by widespread democratic evaluation (Lane, 1995).

The special case of disabled women emphasizes this control in a
particularly poignant way. These women could not avoid the medical
discourse, which has as its core the belief that if there is a risk of
abnormality, or the risk of worsening an already abnormal bodily condition, then steps must be taken to avoid it. Genetic counselling outlining
the "risks," or the option/recommendation of a termination should be
given to those parents who are "at risk" of producing a baby with a serious
impairment. Women with impairments who are "at risk" of worsening their
condition through pregnancy may be advised not to bear children. Management may involve ceasing medication for epilepsy, diabetes, asthma,
mental problems, or reducing or increasing its levels to balance its effects on
the mother and on the infant. Although the majority of nondisabled parents
can take it for granted that the qualities and characteristics of their parenting
are their own decision, disabled women feel under surveillance as incapable
of parenting unless they can prove otherwise (Thomas, 1997).

These lines of reasoning are rejected by some as disablist, social
barriers that restrict activity in bearing children and in being seen as a fit
parent. Disability is a form of social exclusion and not a product of
impairment per se. Although prospective parents should be aware of the
risks and benefits of childbearing, nonreflective patient education can
easily reinforce attitudes of exclusion and incompetence instead of empowering these women to succeed (Thomas, 1997).

The 1980s and 1990s saw antenatal education come under institutional control and away from the influences of the women's and consumer
movements that began in 1960. In some instances, classes are used as

institutional marketing tools. Parents may hear about childbirth the way it is allowed to take place at the sponsoring hospital rather than learn about all options that may be available. Some suggest that core curriculum standards would be helpful in improving quality and avoiding what could be perceived as institutional conflict of interest (Zwelling, 1996). The goals of antenatal education should be building self-efficacy to enable parents to make choices and take control over childbearing and childrearing. The scope of educational offerings for expectant parents has expanded to include preconception, early pregnancy, exercise, cesarean preparation, breastfeeding, newborn care, and infant cardiopulmonary resuscitation, as well as the traditional classes for prepared childbirth. Access to these services by inner-city and rural populations should be improved (Nolan, 1997).

Current health practice has frequently been shown to differ by social variables such as race and socioeconomic status. There is evidence that this is also true with antenatal education. The dangers of maternal health risk behaviors (such as smoking, alcohol consumption, and illegal drug use) during pregnancy have been well documented. Uncorroborated self-reports describe White women of higher socioeconomic status receiving more prenatal advice from health care providers on alcohol and smoking cessation during the first trimester when cessation of these behaviors could lower their risk of an adverse reproductive outcome. Advice on illegal drug use was skewed toward single, less educated, younger, and poorer women. Kogan, Kotelchuck, Alexander, and Johnson (1994) conclude that advice about prenatal health behavior is not a uniform feature of all prenatal care and that it may contribute to differential rates of birth outcomes by race.

A second study (Zambrana, Scrimshaw and Dunkel-Schetter, 1996) shows that African American women are less likely than women of Mexican origin to report being informed and given advice about medical risk conditions. Even though approximately 20% of low-income ethnic women are at medical risk, less than a quarter of both groups of women reported they were given advice.

Education plays an important role at every stage—planning and confirming a pregnancy, prenatal testing, self-care throughout pregnancy, monitoring for preterm labor and postpartum.

PRENATAL CARE AND TESTING

Prenatal testing is now a significant learning experience for increasing numbers of parents, but also with the potential of increased anxiety over

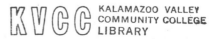

the entire pregnancy. A study by Oliver and others (1996) of providing leaflets to patients summarizing the best available evidence about ultrasonography in early pregnancy provides an interesting case study. The pamphlets reviewed the value of routine scanning in detecting fetal malformations and multiple pregnancies and in estimating gestational age, and discussed the evidence about safety. The leaflet for professionals concluded that ultrasound scanning should not be presented as routine but rather as one possible course of action and recommended offering women an informed choice about whether to have a scan. Ultrasonographers, however, were outraged at this approach, including the communication to the women of potential negative effects of the scan.

Thornton, Hewison, Lilford, and Vail (1995) found that provision of additional information beyond that given routinely about ultrasonography, yielded improved understanding, satisfaction, and decreased anxiety. One possible reason for anxiety in prenatal testing is that patients are frequently unfamiliar with the distinction between a screening and diagnostic test. Pretest patient education is important to enhance patient understanding, control, and decision making and can result in more effective genetic counseling when patients are faced with an abnormal result. Unresolved anxiety during pregnancy in relation to antenatal diagnosis may delay attachment to the pregnancy and infant (Ormond, Pergament, & Fine, 1996).

Concern about attaining adequate patient understanding may be well founded. Freda, DeVore, Valentine-Adams, Bombard, and Merkatz (1998) note that only a few published studies have evaluated what women understand about pregnancy tests in general or maternal serum alpha-fetoprotein (MSAFP) screening in particular. Their study of inner-city minority pregnant women showed that even after instruction, 16% believed something had to be "taken from my belly" for the test. Seventy-two percent thought their infant would be healthy in all respects if the test was negative. Others thought MSAFP could detect drugs taken by the pregnant woman. Although these women had given informed consent for the test and understood it was voluntary, their understanding of the meaning and implications of positive test results was of concern. But what actually constitutes understanding of a subject as complex as MSAFP testing? There is no national standard for informed consent, and courts have not required a specific amount of understanding on the part of patients. The general standards of knowing which treatment is being recommended, its risks and benefits and alternatives does not provide sufficient guidance.

The Maternal Serum Screening Knowledge Questionnaire (MSSKQ) (Table 4.1) has been developed to assess knowledge and provide a focus

TABLE 4.1 MSSKQ Item-Specific and Domain Scores

Question	Intervention group scores (Glazier) n = 133	Scores (Goel) n = 1075	Glazier Controls n = 64
Domain: test characteristics	−.81	1.01	.64*
If maternal serum screening is abnormal, further tests are needed to tell if anything is wrong	1.17	1.11	.92
Maternal serum screening (also called alpha plus or triple test) detects only Down syndrome	.86	1.00	.56*
If maternal serum screening is abnormal, something is usually wrong with the baby	.53	1.05	.64*
Women who have normal maternal serum screening can be sure that they will have a normal baby	.69	.90	.46*
Domain: indications and timing	.64	.91	.73*
Maternal serum screening is not accurate when done at the wrong time during the pregnancy	.72	1.00	.67*
Having maternal serum screening is routine for all pregnant women	.55	.83	.80
Domain: ancillary tests	.53	.89	.32*
Ultrasound can be used to detect every kind of birth defect	.86	1.21	.59*
Amniocentesis can cause miscarriage in about 1 out of 200 women	.75	1.11	.55*
Amniocentesis is a test of the mother's blood which can detect Down syndrome	−.04	.36	.22*
Domain: target conditions	.48	.77	.48*
The chance of having Baby with Down syndrome is higher the older the mother	.96	1.22	.65*
Open neural tube defects include spina bifida (an opening in the bones around the spinal cord) and anencephaly (missing much of the skull and brain)	.75	1.11	.92
All children born with Down syndrome have severe physical and mental disabilities which require life-long care in an institution	.61	.89	.72
If amniocentesis shows Down syndrome, the only options are to have a baby with Down syndrome or to end the pregnancy	.32	.37	.36
The chance of having an open neural tube defect is higher the older the mother	−.28	.29	−.23*
Overall Score	Not reported	.89	.52*

*Significant difference between Glazier intervention and control group of at least .01.

for intervention. Review of educational materials, the literature, and expert opinion was used to reflect information believed to be important for women prior to testing and therefore to reflect content validity. The reading level is equivalent to grade 8. The MSSKQ was pretested and then administered to more than a thousand women, primarily of high socioeconomic status. Internal consistency was .74.

Each item is recorded so that a value of 2 is assigned if the correct response is given with a strongly agree or strongly disagree and a value of 1 assigned for a correct response with merely an agree or disagree statement. Incorrect responses are assigned a value of −2 and −1, respectively and a value of 0 is assigned for a "not sure" response. The score is the average of the scores on each of the 14 items. Scores between −2 and 0 are likely due to incorrect understanding of the information, scores greater than 0 but less than .5 indicate low level of knowledge, and those greater than 1 indicate a high level of knowledge (Glazier et al., 1997; Goel et al., 1996).

Glazier and others (1997) tested an educational pamphlet on triple-marker screening and found that scores on the MSSKQ were significantly higher among the 133 women receiving the intervention pamphlet than among 64 women who received a control pamphlet. The intervention pamphlet was not, however, useful for women who did not speak English at home. The MSSKQ was thus shown to be sensitive to intervention. It can be used to identify specific areas for which knowledge is lacking among groups and individuals.

Educated and informed consent has been seen as an essential component in the offer of prenatal screening due to the complex moral choices that a positive test result can entail. Yet, studies have reported low levels of knowledge about testing among women who have received patient-educational materials, and research on how to best inform pregnant women about genetic tests and their special ethical entailments remains sparse. This issue is particularly acute in California where since 1986 providers have been required to offer alpha fetoprotein (AFP) screening to all women who begin prenatal care before their 20th week of pregnancy. The amount of AFP in the maternal blood at certain stages of pregnancy has been associated with genetic variations and other developmental anomalies in the fetus. Initial positive results can exceed 10% and must be followed by ultrasound and in many cases amniocentesis, for definitive diagnosis. Yet, there is no treatment for virtually all the conditions for which the AFP test screens (Browner, Preloran, & Press, 1996).

Browner et al (1996) found that women who had received an informational booklet and viewed a video about AFP-screening remembered more about the test and its purposes than did those given only the booklet. But what all women remembered most was the procedural information—that it was a voluntary blood test administered during a specific interval but not its purposes or the conditions for which the test screened. Recent Mexican immigrants retained the least information, perhaps in part because the concept of prenatal care is virtually absent in traditional Mexican culture and immigrants to the United States who enroll in prenatal care are often vague about why they have done so.

The informed consent process for genetic counseling can be deficient in a number of ways. The process should involve the health professional explaining the nature of the procedure, its risks, benefits, and alternatives. Once the patient is informed she must be allowed to decide in a noncoerced way whether to undergo the testing. Patients may be given inadequate or misleading information. A physician's own personality and beliefs may influence whether patients are given information about genetic testing in the first place. Some physicians test patients without their consent and pass genetic information on to employers or other third parties. After test results become available, the tested individual may face risks and decisions that are rarely described in the informed-consent process (Andrews, 1997).

So, methods for helping all women understand prenatal screening are urgently needed. Couples who had obtained positive or unfavorable prenatal diagnoses were conflicted about its usefulness (Sandelowski & Jones, 1996). Participants terminating pregnancies believed this foreknowledge saved their babies and themselves from further and/or future suffering. Others believed they could adjust to the news of an impairment during pregnancy and set it aside after birth in favor of bonding to and caring for the baby. Different prenatal tests have different sensitivities and specificities at different stages of pregnancy for different impairments, causing results to be seen later as accurate or inaccurate (false positive or false negative). The knowledge can be difficult to interpret and the options limited (pregnancy termination or continuation with more frequent monitoring, early delivery in a tertiary setting). Foreknowledge can interrupt the presumption of normality, interfere with the pleasure of pregnancy, and create anxiety.

PRETERM LABOR SYMPTOMS

Preterm birth, which occurs in 11% of all pregnancies, is responsible for the majority of neonatal deaths and for other disability. Although all

TABLE 4.2 Symptoms of Preterm Labor

☐ Uterine contractions, every 10 minutes or less, with or without pain
☐ Menstrual-like cramps
☐ Low, dull backache
☐ Pelvic pressure
☐ Changes in vaginal discharge
☐ Urinary frequency
☐ Intestinal cramping with or without diarrhea

From Moore, M. L., & Freda, M. C. (1998). Reducing preterm & low birth-weight births: Still a nursing challenge. *Maternal–Child Nursing, 23,* 200–208. Copyright © 1998 Lippincott, Williams & Wilkins. Reprinted by permission.

births before 37 weeks of gestation are considered premature, births before 32 weeks of gestation account for most neonatal deaths and disorders. The incidence of preterm birth has risen over the past 15% years and remains twice as high among Black women as among White women (Goldenberg & Rouse, 1998).

All pregnant women should be educated about the symptoms of preterm labor, just as all are educated about appropriate nutrition or the avoidance of drugs in pregnancy. Research has shown that women with preterm labor symptoms frequently do not seek care, primarily because they do not understand the importance of the symptoms. Targeting only those considered to be at high risk would miss about half of the women who will ultimately deliver preterm. It is recommended that teaching be simple and direct. Any woman with a pregnancy of 20 to 37 weeks with uterine contractions that do not go away should be concerned and follow the directions in Tables 4.2 and 4.3 (Moore & Freda, 1998).

Freston and others (1997) report as many as a third of women in their

TABLE 4.3 What to Do If Preterm Labor Symptoms Appear

☐ Empty bladder.
☐ Lie down on left side for 1 hour.
☐ Drink two to three large glasses of water or juice.
☐ Palpate for contractions.
☐ If symptoms continue, call health care provider or go to the hospital.
☐ If symptoms stop, resume light activity.
☐ If symptoms reappear, call health care provider or go to the hospital.

From Moore, M. L., & Freda, M. C. (1998). Reducing preterm & low birth-weight births: Still a nursing challenge. *Maternal–Child Nursing, 23,* 200–208. Copyright © 1998 Lippincott, Williams & Wilkins. Reprinted by permission.

study group of healthy well-educated women selected responses to preterm labor symptom questions that would have delayed entry into care. Nine percent believed that menstrual-like cramping was normal, 26% that vaginal discharge was normal, and 19% that backache was normal. Many expressed the belief that as long as contractions were painless, cervical dilitation did not occur, and frequently misinterpreted contractions for fetal movement. Multiparas were not necessarily better at recognizing contractions.

Patients instructed in early detection of premature labor contractions varied greatly in their ability to detect them. Faustin's study (Faustin, Klein, Spector, & Nelson, 1997) showed that 9% of at-risk women consistently failed to detect the contractions even after training and repeated monitoring sessions. The 54% of the population that almost always detects the symptoms of preterm labor should not require monitoring in the absence of complaint. Those in the intermediate category require intermittent monitoring. It is unclear why some women seem unsuccessful in learning to differentiate whether they are in preterm labor. Yet, ability to identify those who can should free them from routine use of the tocodynamometer (Faustin et al., 1997).

An optimal combination of patient education and monitoring to prevent preterm birth is still not clear. In a large study of culturally diverse, well-educated women, Dyson and others (1998) found that neither daily contact with a nurse nor home monitoring of uterine activity provided additional benefit in preventing preterm delivery, as compared with education, daily uterine self-palpation, and weekly contact.

In a review of medical progress in prevention of premature birth, Goldenberg and Rouse (1998) conclude that most interventions designed to prevent preterm birth do not work and the few that do, including treatment of urinary tract infections, cerclage, and treatment of bacterial vaginosis in high-risk women, are applicable to only a small percentage of women at risk for premature birth. The range of interventions that may be seen appears in Table 4.4. The judged lack of effectiveness includes interventions based on patient education, weekly evaluation for signs of preterm labor, and earlier use of tocolytic (labor-inhibiting) therapy.

OTHER ELEMENTS OF PRENATAL EDUCATION

Full plans for prenatal education are well described elsewhere (Sherwen, Scoloveno & Weingarten, 1995). A meta-analysis of prenatal smoking-

TABLE 4.4   Interventions to Prevent Premature Birth

Prenatal care (routine or enhanced)
Risk-scoring systems
Cervical cerclage
Progestin supplementation
Programs for cessation of tobacco, drug, and alcohol use
Psychological support
Nutritional interventions
   Counseling
   Caloric supplementation
   Protein supplementation
   Vitamin or mineral supplementation
Patient education (to detect signs of preterm labor)
Home uterine-activity monitoring
Frequent contact with a nurse
Tocolytic therapy
Bed rest
Hydration
Screening for and treatment of infection (urinary tract infection or bacterial vaginosis)
Antibiotics for preterm labor or premature rupture of membranes
Low-dose aspirin
Calcium supplementation

From Goldenberg, R. L., & Rouse, D. J. (1998). Prevention of premature birth. *New England Journal of Medicine, 339,* 313–320. Copyright © 1998 Massachusetts Medical Society. Reprinted with permission. All rights reserved.

cessation interventions found a 50% increase in smoking cessation (Mullen, Ramirez & Groff, 1994), which is important because maternal smoking is an important cause of low birth weight.

Some excellent examples of cultural ways of approaching others for learning are available. Affonso, Mayberry, Inaba, Matsuno, and Robinson (1996) describe native Hawiian women as dissatisfied with lack of psychosocial help in standard prenatal services, afraid to ask questions for fear of reprimand or criticism, and unclear about what to discuss with their health care providers. Talking about personal issues associated with pregnancy was viewed as inappropriate for this relationship. Prenatal care programs were poorly attended because too many unrealistic expectations were placed on women. A "talk story" used story telling to learn new skills and deal with emotional distress. It provided an opportunity for each woman to share what she believed to be important for her care during pregnancy.

Women wove selected parts of other women's stories into a group cognitive rehearsal, thereby gaining the pooled support and strength from the content of many stories and decreasing feelings of isolation in their fears and expectations. The women articulated their own solutions rather than relying on health providers for answers. After initiation of this culturally appropriate learning intervention there was a vast improvement in prenatal attendance by women in the community (Affonso, Mayberry, Inaba, Matsuno, & Robinson, 1996).

Women decide which pregnancy-related self-care recommendations to accept and which to ignore. Although they see being informed as primary to the responsibilities conferred by pregnancy, many are skeptical about the validity of biomedical information because of the speed with which it has changed. Advice that brought about the promised physiological results was frequently adopted by women in Browner and Press's (1996) study. The women rejected biomedical recommendations they could not easily incorporate into their ongoing daily life circumstances. But they generally deferred to biomedical authority in those domains of prenatal care in which clinical technologies predominate, especially during labor. In reality, much of prenatal care can be seen as a process of medical socialization in which providers attempt to teach pregnant women their own interpretation of the signs and symptoms the women will experience as the pregnancy proceeds and the significance that should be attached to them.

Those who teach patients should understand that the patients must do the work of integrating the advice they are given with their own sense of what is useful. A goal of absolute compliance to all medical advice is not only unreasonable, it also flies in the face of patient informed consent and the integration of the pregnancy into their cultural circle.

One of the goals of prenatal education is to develop the patient's sense of self-efficacy in dealing with labor pain. Relaxation training, distraction, use of imagery, breathing, and other techniques have been shown to have potential particularly in combination, for pain modulation. About half of a group of British women who attempted to put this teaching into practice during labor reported that they were unsuccessful. Many who had attended antenatal classes did not feel "in control" throughout childbirth. Although it is difficult to prepare every woman for the varied and unpredictable experience of childbirth, teaching strategies might be strengthened. Because practice in class is separated in time from use of the skills during labor and the skills have not been practiced under realistic conditions, education concurrent with the pain experience is likely necessary. It is crucial to establish the effectiveness of the coping strategies that are taught in modulating the pain of childbirth (Niven & Gijsbers, 1996).

POSTPARTUM EDUCATION

Postnatal care of women has been said to be relatively neglected as the focus is on the infant. Several studies have shown that health problems are common in women during this time and that many do not seek professional help and have not been taught realistic expectations and self-care activities. Half of women in a British study experienced postnatal sexual problems (Glazener, 1997). In an Australian study, one or more health problems in the first 6 postnatal months were reported by 94% of women; a quarter had not talked to a health professional about their own health since the birth. Half would have liked more help or advice. Most common was tiredness, backache, sexual problems, hemorrhoids, perineal pain, and depression (Brown & Lumley, 1998). Fecal incontinence as an immediate consequence of childbirth has been found to be more common (6%, with a mean duration of 23 weeks) than previously thought, and medical attention was rarely sought. These problems are underreported and underrecognized, and ones with which women seem to cope silently (MacArthur, Bick & Keighley, 1997). Teaching programs should address them.

The scope of educational offerings for expectant parents has expanded to include preconception, early pregnancy, exercise, cesarean preparation, breast-feeding, newborn care, infant cardiopulmonary resuscitation, and parenting classes, as well as the traditional classes for prepared childbirth (Zwelling, 1996).

A very interesting learning process occurs as mothers gain knowledge about and develop a relationship with their babies through perceiving and interpreting their babies' behavior and responses. Mothers must adapt these skills to include the changes consistent with normally and possibly abnormally developing babies. This is a complex process. Identifying what their babies' needs, actions, and responses mean is a major process of learning. Mothers believed that babies sent precise signals to them, and they had a responsibility to learn what these signals meant. Action to alleviate the baby's discomfort is taken while trying to identify the cause that is sometimes never identified. Mothers continued to try to identify the problem until the baby signaled that the problem was over. Although mothers are challenged to care for the needs of each new baby regardless of previous infant-care experience, multiparas have a repertoire for soothing techniques to meet or prevent cries from developing or escalating. These women learned from others who had experience, listening for information that was specific to their babies' circumstances. A patient-education approach that supports and extends this type of learning is a welcome complement to task-oriented education (Sullivan, 1997).

These skills are especially important when infants and mothers have special needs. Mothers of infants were more inaccurate when discriminating causes of low-birth weight premature (LBPW) infant cries and more apt to withdraw from cries of these babies than to respond to them. These effects do not seem to lessen over time, as mothers of LBPW infants 6 months old were not better than those with LBWP newborns at judging cries. Presumably, teaching interventions could help mothers gain control, decrease guilt and uncertainty, and increase self-confidence. Such effects are important as these mother–infant dyads continue to be high risk for several months after leaving the hospital (Worchel & Allen, 1997).

Brooten and others' (1996) study of nursing care of special-needs infants documents the heavy teaching demands. For example, in early discharge after unplanned cesarean birth, assessment of mothers' learning needs surrounding their ability to assume self-care and care of newborn included: understanding signs and symptoms of maternal and newborn infection, limitations on physical activity, maternal and newborn dietary needs, normal bowel function, amount and duration of expected vaginal bleeding, and resumption of sexual activity. The nurse specialist also evaluated the woman's coping ability, support systems, and perceived needs for convalesence and parenting. More than half of the women required more than two home visits as well as phone calls. Current health care services that may provide one or two 1-hour home visits to childbearing women at high risk may not be meeting the education and resource needs of this group. Failure to address the teaching and other needs of patients discharged early may result in increased acute care visits and hospital readmittance, with the associated health care costs.

Another special group is teenage mothers. Deficits in knowledge of child development and unrealistic expectations of children's abilities are often cited as problems for these mothers. Recent research has documented that adult mothers had greater knowledge of infant development than did adolescent mothers. For both groups, social support and knowledge of infant development were significantly correlated with confidence in providing infant care, although this knowledge was found to be an especially important factor in maternal confidence for adolescents (Ruchala & James, 1997).

Other postpartum teaching needs affect many new mothers. In postpartum blues, a transitory state appears in up to 85% of all new mothers 2–4 days postpartum and lasting no more than 2 weeks. Typical symptoms include tearfulness, mood lability, irritability, and anxiety. Reassurance, support, and education are sufficient in most cases. Those conditions that are more serious (postpartum depression and postpartum psychosis) must be differentiated. These disorders can disrupt family life, have a negative effect on development of the infant and increase the risk of subsequent psychopathology in the mother. Rates of postpartum depression appear lower in cultures where women receive assistance, appreciation of their new roles as mothers, education about the techniques of mothering, and an opportunity to rest following delivery (Burt & Hendrick, 1997). At 2 weeks postpartum, Fishbein and Burggraf (1998) found 25% of respondents to their study indicating they were depressed or experiencing the "baby blues."

Teaching and support for breast-feeding is a major commitment of some health professionals. Lactation specialists and clinics specializing in this service are available but have had to accomodate to short hospital stays. Sleepy infants, lack of maternal psychological readiness, and lack of full milk supply make early education difficult. Recognizing early hunger cues such as rooting, sucking, and hand-to-mouth motor behavior are important, as crying is the last hunger cue and signals frantic hungriness. Table 4.5 outlines a care map for breast-feeding. Sucking is not considered a reassuring sign; swallowing is the key. Swallowing is frequently underemphasized in textbooks and patient-education materials. Unless successful feeding has been observed and documented postpartum, one cannot presume that it will eventually occur after discharge. Teaching parents to monitor symptoms of dehydration is important, as is recognition of early signs of jaundice (Biancuzzo, 1997).

Table 4.6 is an example of a written teaching tool addressing prevention and care of sore nipples (Bell & Rawlings, 1998). Women should be assisted to a comfortable position and shown how to support the breast in a cupped hand with the thumb on top and fingers underneath. This promotes an optimal deep latching position for the baby. As the care map indicates, mothers should be assisted to stimulate the baby's wide-open mouth. Practice will help the mother bring the baby onto the breast so that the gums latch with an inch to inch and a half of areola behind the nipple in the mouth (Bell & Rawlings, 1998). These skills should be learned through demonstration and practice to the point of proficiency and confidence.

There is evidence that many providers supply incorrect information about breast-feeding to families. Education has been shown to improve initiation and duration of breast-feeding among various populations. Many advocate promoting human lactation as a preventive health practice that should come as easily to health professionals as recommending that infant car seats be used or cautioning pregnant women about the risks of

TABLE 4.5   Care Map for Breast-Feeding

Signal	Before 24 hr	24–48 hr	48–72 hr
Alertness	Alert sometimes	Alert most times	Alert for all feedings
Alignment	Mom correctly aligns infant in one or two positions with assistance.	Mom correctly aligns infant in one position independently; aligns infant in two to three positions with help.	Mom correctly aligns infant for three positions independently.
Areolar grasp	Mom verbalizes importance of *open wide.*	Mom is reassured by open wide.	Baby consistently opens wide.
Areolar compression	Mom identifies difference in sucking patterns (nonnutritive versus nutritive sucking).	Infant exhibits long, slow, rhythmic sucks at most feedings.	Infant exhibits long, slow rhythmic sucks at all feedings.
Audible swallowing	Mom verbalizes importance of audible swallowing.	Infant audibly swallows.	Infant audibly swallows.
Frequency/ milk supply	Mom feeds/stimulates every 2 to 3 hours.	Mom feeds/stimulates every 2 to 3 hours.	Mom feeds/ stimulates every 2 to 3 hours.

Source: Reprinted with permission from M. Biancuzzo, *Breastfeeding the Neonate: Clinical Strategies for Nurses.* Copyright © 1999 C.V. Mosby Co.

drinking alcohol and smoking (Bell & Rawlings, 1998). The focus of such education should instead be on providing full information to assist an informed decision by the woman/couple.

Human immunodeficiency virus (HIV) can be transmitted to the infant through breast milk, and some drugs such as antineoplastics, lithium, and others are contraindications to breast-feeding (Thureen & Hay, 1996). Because support of the father is frequently critical to successful breast-feeding, education should include helping fathers develop infant-comforting skills, self-efficacy in relating with the infant, and knowledge about breast-feeding (Sharma & Petosa, 1997).

Motivational education to promote breast-feeding is described in a couple of studies of economically disadvantaged women. In one setting (Libbus, 1994) all prenatal clients were expected to attend breast-feed-

TABLE 4.6   Preventing and Caring for Sore Nipples

Breast-feeding should not be painful!
Some tenderness during the first few seconds of nursing is normal and generally goes away in a week to 10 days. The nipples shouldn't be cracked, blistered, bleeding, or so sore that the pain makes you cry. If you feel that much pain or have those symptoms, ask your health care provider for help.

The best way to prevent sore nipples is to be sure the baby is positioned properly and latches on the breast I correctly.

Get comfortable. Have good back support and extra pillows to support your arms and one in your lap. A small foot stool provides welcome support under your feet.

Use Various Positions
You may nurse in many different positions. Sometimes it helps to change nursing positions to drain one part of the breast more completely or to ease the pain on one part of the nipple.

In any position, your baby should face you so that his/her head, neck, and body are in line. The baby shouldn't have to turn his/her head to nurse.

Football/Clutch Position
This position is often easiest for new mothers and babies. Position your baby facing you and tucked under your arm. Have a pillow or two next to you to help support the baby and your arm. Support your baby's head and neck with your hand, allowing your forearm to support his/her body against the side of yours.

Cradle Position
This position works well for older babies. Place one or two pillows in your lap to help support the baby. His/her head will be in the crook of your arm. Turn baby's body to face you, tummy to tummy. Your opposite hand supports your breast.

Side-Lying Position
Lie on your side with pillows supporting your back, neck, and head. Place another pillow between your legs. Try bending your top leg forward. Position the baby on his/her side, facing you.

Support the Breast Throughout the Feeding
Support your breast by cupping it with one of your hands, positioning the fingers and thumb well back from the areola (brownish part of the nipple). Your thumb will be on top of the breast and your other fingers below the breast, forming the letter C.

If you don't support the breast, at least during the early days of nursing, gravity causes the breast to pull the nipple forward in the baby's mouth, allowing him to suck on the end of the nipple. This position can cause pain, bruising, and cracking of the skin over or around the nipple. Supporting your breast also helps to keep the nipple deep in the baby's mouth to stimulate sucking.

TABLE 4.6 (Continued)

Stimulate Your Baby to Open Wide
Stroke your baby's face from nose to chin until he opens his mouth wide. Then quickly bring him to breast with the arm and hand supporting him. As his mouth closes, his tongue should remain over his lower gum line.

Ask someone to help you by making sure the baby's bottom lip is flared outward as he nurses. His nose should touch the breast. The baby's mouth should contain the nipple and about an inch to an inch and a half of the areola. Support your breast throughout the feeding.

Nurse Your Baby Frequently
Newborns need to nurse every 1½ to 3 hours, or about 8 to 12 times every 24 hours. Most need to nurse 10 to 20 minutes on each breast during the early days. *Limiting the frequency of feedings can make sore nipples worse.* Infrequent feedings lead to engorged breasts, making correct latching-on difficult for the baby. A frantically hungry baby may not latch or suck well, causing further damage to the nipple.

Break the Suction Gently
Place a clean finger between his gums to release the suction before taking him off the breast. You will feel his mouth release the breast.

After Nursing
At the end of a feeding, express a little colostrum or milk and rub it into your nipple and areola. Allow the area to air dry. Human milk contains antibodies that fight infection. The milk also contains fat, which acts as a skin moisturizer.

Nipple Care
You don't have to wash your breasts before or after a feeding. Showering or bathing once a day will keep your breasts clean. Never use soap, alcohol, or baby wipes on your breasts or nipples; they have a drying effect.

Change nursing pads as soon as they become moist. Never use pads or bras with plastic liners.

Using a pure USP-modified lanolin cream or ointment can be soothing. Apply it sparingly to your nipples after they have been air-dried.

Taking Care of Sore Nipples
Make sure your baby is latching onto the breast and sucking properly so that no further damage is done to your sore nipples. If you aren't sure the baby is latched on well, call your health care provider or lactation consultant for an evaluation.

Vary the positions in which you nurse.

Nurse on the less painful side first.

(continued)

TABLE 4.6 (Continued)

Limit nursing time to about 10 minutes on the affected breast or on both sides if both nipples are sore. Once the soreness has faded, you won't have to limit the baby's time at the breast.

After nursing, express a little colostrum or milk and rub it into the nipple and areola. Do this after nursing and, if you are very sore, every hour. Follow with air-drying for 5 to 10 minutes.

Allow the skin to air-dry; then apply a very small amount of a USP-modified lanolin to your nipples after nursing.

Don't wear nipple shields during feedings. Nipple shells, worn between feedings, may allow air to circulate around sore nipples. They also prevent clothing and nursing pads from sticking to tender skin. Bathe nipples with 1 tablespoon of vinegar in 1 cup of water or 1 teaspoon of baking soda in 1 cup of water, followed by air-drying.

Call your health care provider if:
- Pain and tenderness continue for 7 to 10 days or more.
- A crack or blister on the nipple doesn't heal in 7 to 10 days.
- You feel a burning pain at the nipple or inside the breast during and between feedings.
- You feel itching and burning pain at the nipple.
- Your nipples are painful and bright pink or red.

Used with permission from K. K. Bell & N. L. Rowlings: Promoting Breast-feeding by Managing Common Lactation Problems. *The Nurse Practitioner, 23*(6): 102–123. Springhouse Corporation. Copyright © Springhouse Corporation.

ing classes, regardless of stated feeding choice. Gross and others (1998) report a series of 8 trigger video vignettes, each 2 to 5 minutes in length, that addressed the benefits and major barriers to breast-feeding to African American women attending Special Supplemental Nutrition Program for Women, Infants, and Children (WIC) clinics. Posters, pamphlets, and counseling sessions were also used. The videos were played in the waiting area. A peer counselor assessed the women's attitudes regarding infant feeding, corrected misconceptions, held counseling or group support sessions on infant feeding, dropped off a breast-feeding promotional gift package postpartum, and confirmed follow-up plans. After delivery peer counselors attempted to contact breast-feeding women biweekly to address any problems or questions related to infant feeding. All peer counselors were present or former WIC clients, had successfully breast-fed at least one child, and had completed a 5–week training program.

Women in the intervention clinics were about one third less likely to stop breast-feeding before 16 weeks postpartum compared with women in the control group, which was provided with nutrition education and breast-feeding promotion activities. One has to ask where the line is between promotion of or manipulation into breast feeding, especially as poor minority women were targeted for the interventions.

Mothers who choose breast-feeding do so largely for the benefits to the baby, perhaps in part because this is what is emphasized in prenatal teaching. Benefits to the mother are rarely emphasized but include protection from hemorrhage through release of oxytocin with every feeding, delay in return of menses and therefore of fertility with regular breast-feeding, and loss and maintenance of weight loss (Dermer, 1998).

No matter what their chosen infant-feeding method, mothers need to master a number of infant-feeding skills: positioning for latch-on and comfort, bottle cleaning, formula preparation, reception and interpretation of cues from the infant, use of a breast pump, knowledge of when infants are getting enough, and of how to combine breast-feeding and bottle feeding.

PARENTING OF INFANTS AND CHILDREN

There are many examples of education for mothering. Confidence in one's ability as a fully responsible caregiver has to be developed, as does problem-solving skill and satisfaction as a parent (Pridham, 1997). The multiple examples that follow show how great the need is and how important the interventions.

Mothering of preterm infants should begin with a specific and ongoing role in the care of the infant in the hospital, which has been shown to improve parenting. Interaction patterns developed at this time affect later interactions and caregiving. Prematurity continues to affect parenting in the preschool period (Holditch-Davis & Miles, 1997). A prospective, longitudinal study of low-birthweight, preterm infants found a small but significant effect of maternal knowledge and concepts of child development and quality of the home environment and number of child behavior problems. The effect of maternal knowledge was apparent by the time the child was 12 months of age (Benasich & Brooks-Gunn, 1996).

Sometimes mothers don't seem to have the information they need or

TABLE 4.7   Knowledge About Otitis Media

Question (correct response)	Percentage
Drainage coming from the ear may be a sign of ear infection. (T)	87
Children are most likely to get ear infections between 3 and 5 years of age. (F)	86
Taking babies outside without caps or hats can cause ear infections. (F)	65
Babies often have ear infections without any sign they are sick. (T)	78
Babies who are cared for at home are just as likely to get ear infections as babies who attend day care centers. (F)	35
During the winter taking babies outside with wet hair can lead to ear infections. (F)	65
Ear infections tend to run in families. (T)	50
Formula-fed babies and breastfed babies tend to have the same number of ear infections. (F)	65
Ear infections can affect a baby's hearing. (T)	96
Most ear infections get better by themselves. (T)	11
A baby is likely to get an ear infection when a new tooth is coming in. (F)	60

Reproduced with permission from *Pediatrics,* vol. 100, pages 931–936. 1997.

to act on it. Even though otitis media (OM) is the most common diagnosis for children under 2 years of age in the United States, studies in Minnesota show lack of knowledge about risk factors. Misunderstandings as well as areas of correct knowledge may be found in Table 4.7. Potentially modifiable risk factors for OM (such as day-care attendance, smoking, and lack of breast-feeding), were prevalent among these Minnesota infants during their first year of life, a period when OM incidence is high. Only a quarter of the mothers in this study reported receiving information about OM prevention (Daly, Selvius, & Lindgren, 1997).

In another example, low-income African American mothers of children with sickle cell disease (SCD) studied by Hill (1994a, 1994b) rejected or redefined the medical model that the course and severity of the disease is unpredictable, that SCD was serious and incurable, and could be eliminated only through genetic screening and selective mating. The medical model assumes that persons with the trait will alter their reproductive behavior to avoid having a child with the disease. This model has not offered a viable and coherent strategy to manage the disease.

Mothers were not interested in learning medicine's knowledge about the origin and transmission of SCD; instead, they focused on firsthand experientially acquired knowledge about how to cope with the disease. They placed high priority on their reproductive autonomy to become mothers, and many knew they had the trait prior to having a child with the disease.

The mothers in this study were among the first generation of U. S. Blacks to receive widespread education and testing for SCD but were also victimized by the misinformation and erroneous diagnoses that characterized the early SCD screening efforts. These mothers knew of the racial politics and believed that the medical system could not be trusted to handle a race-specific disease.

From a critical perspective, White, male authorities are deciding which diseases constitute unacceptable health risk. SCD screening programs place the onus of responsibility for controlling the disease on women because they are more likely than men to be screened for a genetic trait, to use birth control, and/or make childbearing decisions. These mothers may not have had enough power in their relationships with men to persuade potential fathers to be screened. At any rate, their class and gender positions created barriers to using SCD medical knowledge and their goals were apparently not the same as those of medicine—to prevent the births of children with the disease. This experience demonstrates that education based on a model thought by the target group to be unbelievable frequently cannot overide strong cultural values including those placed on motherhood (Hill, 1994a).

Medicine is a political as well as a scientific field and patient-education programs inevitably reflect that fact. Consider how a patient-education program oriented to the women's perceived needs might differ from the previously dominant patient-education model based on the medical assumptions outlined above.

A fourth example of mothering education concerns the special population of chemically dependent women. The dysfunctional family histories, poor coping skills, inadequate social support networks and negative affective states often experienced by chemically dependent women set them up for being unable to provide optimal parenting to their children, despite their desire to do so. Parenting is believed to be in part a learned behavior from one's family of origin. Parenting education and support services are important components to consider when planning for the recovery needs of these women. These services offer skill and knowledge development on topics such as child development, effective disciplinary techniques, play strategies, and parenting under stress (Davis, 1997).

After they are committed to the recovery process and issues such as depression and anger have been addressed, chemically dependent women need to interact with their children in the presence of professionals who can provide a role model and knowledge and feedback about effective parenting strategies. This includes how to respect children's needs, how to talk so that children will listen, how to establish routines and rituals, and how to set limits that are age appropriate. Being taught how to provide quality playtime with their children is important (Davis, 1997).

Newborn care is another important parenting skill that chemically dependent women often lack, despite having multiple pregnancies. Their newborns may have been taken from them at birth and placed in protective custody because they show signs and symptoms of in utero drug exposure and may be fussy and difficult to comfort. Teaching these women about the health needs of their children is also important. They may be too intimidated to seek care, do not recognize the importance of seeking health care for their children, or appreciate the need to use regular well-child services (Davis, 1997).

A final example describes the Creating Opportunities for Parent Empowerment (COPE) program for mothers of critically ill children. The program recognizes the overwhelming anxiety faced by these mothers and the potential to improve their ability to provide support to their children during intrusive procedures, how to deal with their own stress, and decrease negative behavioral and emotional changes in their children. Parents were educated about: (a) the known behaviors and emotions of hospitalized children, (b) recognition of how parents experience a change in parental role during a child's hospitalization, (c) instruction and practice in parenting behaviors specific to the situation of dealing with a hospitalized child, and (d) maternal understanding about the effects of hospitalization on their children and how it affects the mothers' confidence in their parenting role. Practice is included in the instruction, in order to increase maternal confidence and role certainty. Details of this research-based intervention may be found in Melnyk, Alpert-Gillis, Hensel, Cable-Beiling, and Rubenstein (1997).

MEASUREMENT INSTRUMENTS

A number of measurement tools are available for assessment of mother's need for education and to evaluate its outcome. The tools listed in the box that follows are presented and reviewed in Redman (1998). The Parent Behavior Checklist, developed by Robert Fox, is also reviewed. A review of breast-feeding assessment tools (Riordan & Koehn, 1997) provides citations to three such tools but finds that reliability coefficients for all three are below acceptable levels for clinical decisions. Because early hospital discharge of new mothers makes assessment of breast-feeding skills difficult, the availability of a simple, reliable assessment tool that would also predict breast-feeding problems would be a valuable contribution to the care of mothers and their newborns (Riordan & Koehn, 1997).

Pregnancy Anxiety Scale, developed by Jeffrey Levin
Childbirth Expectations Questionnaire, developed by Annette Gupton
Labour Agentry Scale, developed by Ellen Hodnett
Childbirth Self-Efficacy Inventory, developed by Nancy K. Lowe
Maternal Self-Efficacy Scale, developed by Douglas M. Teti and Donna M. Gelfand
Diabetes in Pregnancy Knowledge Screen, developed by Anthony Spirito, Laurie Ruggerio, Andrea Bond, Lee Rotondo, and Donald R. Coustan
Knowledge of Maternal Phenylketonuria Test, developed by Shoshana Shiloh, Paula St. James, and Susan Waisbren
Parent Expectations Survey, developed by Susan McClennan Reece
Infant Care Survey, developd by Robin D. Froman and Steven V. Owen
How I Deal with Problems Regarding Care of My Baby Questionnaire, developed by Karen F. Pridham and Audrey S. Chang
Toddler Care Questionnaire, developed by Deborah Gross and Lorraine Rocissano

---

Parent Behavior Checklist

The Parent Behavior Checklist (PBC) was developed by Robert Fox; this rating scale measures developmental expectations and reported behaviors of children between the ages of 1 and 4 years, 11 months. Experts and parents of young children rated items developed from the research and clinical literature. Initially known as the Parenting Inventory: Young Children, the PBC has been tested with well over a thousand mothers. In most studies, mothers were selected for study because they continue to take primary responsibility for raising young children.

The PBC is written at a third-grade level. A 4-point rating scale is used with 4 = always/almost always, 3 = frequently, 2 = sometimes and 1 = never/almost never. Higher scores on the Expectations subscale are associated with higher parental expectations, on the Discipline subscale with more frequent use of corporal and verbal punishment, and on the Nurturing subscale with more frequent use of positive nurturing activities like playing and reading (Solis-Camara & Fox, 1995).

Factor analysis showed three scales: Expectations—50 items about parents' developmental expectations (alpha .97, test–retest after 1 week .98); Discipline—30 items that assess parental responses to problem child behaviors (alpha .91, test–retest .87); Nurturing—20 items that measure specific parent behaviors that promote a child's psychological growth (alpha .82, test–retest .81). All three subscales, but especially the expectations subscale, were found to be sensitive to the age of the parent's child. PBC also differentiated from measures of parent attitudes; both of these findings support its validity as does its high correlation with an independent developmental questionnaire. Social desirability did not appear to be a significant factor in mothers' responses on the inventory (Peters & Fox, 1993). Mean scores may be found in Fox and Bentley (1992). Parents of 2- and 3-year-old girls had significantly higher expectations that did parents of boys in the same age ranges.

The PBC has also been used with Mexican mothers and children. Mothers from higher socioeconomic levels in both Mexico and the United States held higher developmental expectations for their children and used less frequent discipline and more frequent nurturing practices than mothers from lower socioeconomic levels (Solis-Camara & Fox, 1995, 1996).

The PBC may be used several ways: identification of parents with unrealistically high expectations for their children, as evaluation for interventions aimed at reducing unreasonable expectations, and inappropriate discipline strategies. Parents who score significantly below the mean may need encouragement to increase their expectations (Fox, 1992; Fox & Bentley, 1992).

SUMMARY

Motherhood provides multiple opportunities for learning and growing, not only in competence in parenting a new child but about oneself. The experiences and learning support needs of some groups seem not to have been addressed by the medical mainstream system or its educational arm. Many have expressed concerns about education that may not include the full range of options or support the autonomy of the mother in making her own informed decisions. A number of useful measurement tools are available in this field, yet there is little evidence of their use in routine clinical practice. Although examples in this chapter have primarily focused on new motherhood, learning needs continue.

REFERENCES

Affonso, D. D., Mayberry, L., Inaba, A., Matsuno, R., & Robinson, E. (1996). Hawaiian-style "Talkstory": psychosocial assessment and intervention during and after pregnancy. *Journal of Obstetric, Gynecologic, and Neonatal Nursing, 25,* 737–742.

Andrews, L. B. (1997). Compromised consent: deficiencies in the consent process for genetic testing. *Journal of the American Medical Women's Association, 52,* 39–44.

Bell, K. K., & Rawlings, N. L. (1998). Promoting breast-feeding by managing common lactation problems. *Nurse Practitioner, 23*(6), 102–123.

Benasich, A. A., & Brooks-Gunn, S. (1996). Maternal attitudes and knowledge of child-rearing: Associations with family and child outcomes. *Child Development, 67,*1186–1205.

Biancuzzo, M. (1997). Breastfeeding education for early discharge: A three-tiered approach. *Journal of Perinatal Neonatal Nursing, 11*(2), 10–22.

Brooten, D., Knapp, H., Borucki, L., Jacobsen, B., Finkler, S., Arnold, L., & Mennuti, M. (1996). Early discharge & home care after unplanned Cesarean birth: Nursing care time. *Journal of Obstetric, Gynecologic, and Neonatal Nursing, 25,* 595–600.

Brown, S., & Lumley, J. (1998). Maternal health after childbirth: Rresults of an Australian population based survey. *British Journal of Obstetrics & Gynaecology, 105,* 156–161.

Browner, C. H., Preloran, M., & Press, N. A. (1996). The effects of ethnicity, education and an informational video on pregnant women's knowledge and decisions about a prenatal diagnostic screening test. *Patient Education & Counseling, 27,* 135–146.

Browner, C. H., & Press, N. (1996). The production of authoritative knowledge in American prenatal care. *Medical Anthropology Quarterly, 10,* 141–156.

Burt, V. K. & Hendrick, V. C. (1997). *Women's mental health.* Washington, DC; American Psychiatric Press.

Daly, K. A., Selvius, R. E., & Lindgren, B. (1997). Knowledge & attitudes about otitis media risk: Implications for prevention. *Pediatrics, 100,* 931–936.

Davis, S. K. (1997). Comprehensive interventions for affecting the parenting effectiveness of chemically dependent women. *Journal of Obstetric, Gynecologic, and Neonatal Nursing, 26,* 604–610.

Dermer, A. (1998). Breastfeeding and women's health. *Journal of Women's Health, 7,* 427–433.

Dyson, D. C., Danbe, K. H., Bamber, J. A., Crites, Y. M., Field, D. R., Maier, J. A., Newman, L. A., Ray, D. A., Walton, D. L., & Armstrong, M. A. (1998). Monitoring women at risk for preterm labor. *New England Journal of Medicine, 338,* 15–19.

Faustin, D., Klein, S., Spector, I. J. & Nelson, J. (1997). Maternal perception of preterm labor: Is it reliable? *Journal of Maternal-Fetal Medicine, 6,* 184–186.

Feitshans, I. L. (1995). Legislating to preserve women's autonomy during pregnancy. *Medicine & Law, 14,* 397–412.

Fishbein, E. G., & Burggraf, E. (1998). Early postpartum discharge: How are mothers managing? *Journal of Obstetric, Gynecologic, and Neonatal Nursing, 27,* 142–148.

Fox, R. A. (1992). Development of an instrument to measure the behaviors & expectations of parents of young children. *Journal of Pediatric Psychology, 17,* 231–239.

Fox, R. A., & Bentley, K. S. (1992). Validity of the Parenting Inventory: Young children. *Psychology in the Schools, 29,* 101–106.

Freda, M. C., DeVore, N., Valentine-Adams, N., Bombard, A., & Merkatz, I. (1998). Informed consent for maternal serum alpha-fetoprotein screening in an inner city population: How informed is it? *Journal of Obstetric, Gynecologic, and Neonatal Nursing, 27,* 99–106.

Freston, M. S., Young, S., Calhoun, S., Fredericksen, T., Salinger, L., Malchodi, C., & Egan, J. F. X. (1997). Responses of pregnant women to potential preterm labor symptoms. *Journal of Obstetric, Gynecologic, and Neonatal Nursing, 26,* 35–41.

Glazener, C. M. A. (1997). Sexual function after childbirth: Women's experiences, presistent morbidity and lack of professional recognition. *British Journal of Obstetrics & Gynecology, 104,* 330–335.

Glazier, R., Goel, V., Holzapfel, S., Summers, A., Pugh, P., & Yeung, M. (1997). Written patient information about triple-marker screening: A randomized controlled trial. *Obstetrics & Gynecology, 90,*769–774.

Goel, V., Glazier, R., Holzapfel, S., Pugh, P., & Summers, A. (1996). Evaluating patient's knowledge of maternal serum screening. *Prenatal Diagnosis, 16,* 425–430.

Goldenberg, R. L., & Rouse, D. J. (1998). Prevention of premature birth. *New England Journal of Medicine, 339,* 313–320.

Gross, S. M., Caulfield, L. E., Bentley, M. E., Bronner, Y., Kessler, L., Jensen, J., & Paige, D. M. (1998). Counseling and motivational videotapes increase duration of breast-feeding in African-American WIC participants who initiate breast-feeding. *Journal of the American Dietetic Association, 98,* 143–148.

Hill, S. A. (1994a). Motherhood & the obfuscation of medical knowledge: The case of sickle cell disease. *Gender & Society, 8,* 29–47.

Hill, S. A. (1994b). *Managing sickle cell disease in low-income families.* Philadelphia: Temple University Press.

Holditch-Davis, D., & Miles, M. S. (1997). Parenting the prematurely born child. In Joyce J. Fitzpatrick & J. Norbeck (Eds.), *Annual review of nursing research* (Vol. 16, pp. 3–34). New York: Springer Publishing Co.

Kogan, M. D., Kotelchuck, M., Alexander, G. R., & Johnson, W. E. (1994). Racial disparities in reported prenatal care advice from health care providers. *American Journal of Public Health, 84,* 82–88.

Lane, K. (1995). The medical model of the body as a site of risk: A case study of childbirth. In J. Gabe (Ed.), *Medicine, health & risk.* Cambridge, MA: Blackwell.

Libbus, M. K. (1994). Lactation education practice and procedure: Information and support offered to economically disadvantaged women. *Journal of Community Health Nursing, 11,* 1–10.

MacArthur, C., Bick, D. E., & Keighley, M. R. B. (1997). Faecal incontinence after childbirth. *British Journal of Obstetrics & Gynaecology, 104,* 46–50.

McVeigh, C. (1997). Motherhood experiences from the perspective of first-time mothers. *Clinical Nursing Research, 6,* 335–348.

Melnyk, B. M., Alpert-Gillis, L. J., Hensel, P. B., Cable-Beiling, R. C., & Rubenstein, J. S. (1997). Helping mothers cope with a critically ill child: A pilot test of the COPE intervention. *Research in Nursing & Health, 20,* 3–14.

Moore, M. L., & Freda, M. C. (1998). Reducing preterm and low birthweight births: Still a nursing challenge. *Maternal–Child Nursing, 23,* 200–208.

Mullen, P. D., Ramirez, G., & Groff, J. Y. (1994). A meta-analysis of randomized trials of prenatal smoking cessation interventions. *American Journal of Obstetrics & Gynecology, 171,* 1328–1334.

Niven, C. A., & Gijsbers, K. (1996). Coping with labor pain. *Journal of Pain & Symptom Management, 11,* 116–125.

Nolan, M. L. (1997). Antenatal education—where next? *Journal of Advanced Nursing, 25,* 1198–1204.

Oliver, S., Rajan, L., Turner, H., Oakley, A., Entwistle, V., Watt, I., Sheldon, T. A., & Rosser, J. (1996). Informed choice for users of health services: Views on ultrasonography leaflets of women in early pregnancy, midwives, and ultrasonographers. *British Medical Journal, 313,*1251–1255.

Ormond, K. E., Pergament, E., & Fine, B. A. (1996). Pre-screening education in multiple marker screening programs: The effect on patient anxiety & knowledge. *Journal of Genetic Counseling, 5,* 69–80.

Peters, C. L., & Fox, R. A. (1993). Parenting Inventory: Validity & social desirability. *Psychological Reports, 72,* 683–689.

Pridham, K. F. (1997). Mothers' help seeking as care initiated in a social context. *Image, 29,* 65–70.

Redman, B. K. (1998). *Measurement tools in patient education.* New York: Springer Publishing Co.

Riordan, J. M., & Koehn, M. (1997). Reliability and validity testing of three breastfeeding assessment tools. *Journal of Obstetric, Gynecologic, and Neonatal Nursing, 26,* 181–187.

Ruchala, P. L., & James, D. C. (1997). Social support, knowledge of infant development, and maternal confidence among adolescent & adult mothers. *Journal of Obstetric, Gynecologic, and Neonatal Nursing, 26,* 685–689.

Sandelowski, M., & Jones, L. C. (1996). Couples' evaluations of foreknowledge of fetal impairment. *Clinical Nursing Research, 5,* 81–96.

Sharma, M., & Petosa, R. (1997). Impact of expectant fathers in breast-feeding decisions. *Journal of the American Dietetic Association, 97,* 1311–1313.

Sherwen, L. N., Scoloveno, M. A., & Weingarten, C. T. (1995). *Nursing care of the childbearing family* (2nd ed.). Norwalk, CT: Appleton & Lange.

Solis-Camara, P., & Fox, R. A. (1995). Parenting among mothers with young children in Mexico & the United States. *Journal of Social Psychology, 135,* 591–599.

Solis-Camara, P., & Fox, R. A. (1996). Parenting practices & expectations among Mexican mothers with young children. *Journal of Genetic Psychology, 157,* 465–476.

Sullivan, J. M. (1997). Learning the baby: A maternal thinking & problem-solving process. *Journal of the Society of Pediatric Nurses, 2,* 21–28.

Thomas, C. (1997). The baby & the bath water: Disabled women and motherhood in social context. *Sociology of Health & Illness, 19,* 622–643.

Thornton, J. G., Hewison, J., Lilford, R. J., & Vail, A. (1995). *British Medical Journal, 311,* 1127–1130.

Thureen, P. J., & Hay, W. W., Jr. (1996). Advice for selected breast-feeding issues. *Comprehensive Therapy, 22,* 802–805.

Worchel, F. F., & Allen, M. (1997). Mothers' ability to discriminate cry types in low-birthweight premature and full-term infants. *Children's Health Care, 26,* 183–195.

Zambrana, R. E., Scrimshaw, S. C. M., & Dunkel-Schetter, C. (1996). Prenatal care and medical risk in low-income, primiparous, Mexican-origin and African American women. *Families, Systems & Health, 14,*349–359.

Zwelling, E. (1996). Childbirth education in the 1990s and beyond. *Journal of Obstetric, Gynecologic, and Neonatal Nursing, 25,* 425–432.

CHAPTER FIVE

Cancer Patient Education

Although heart disease is the leading cause of death and disability for women, cancer is a significant health problem and probably the one that is most feared. Breast cancer is by far the most common cancer among both White (113.2 per 100,000) and Black females (94.0 per 100,000). Lung cancer and colorectal cancer are the second and third highest cancers, respectively, among White females compared to ranks of third and second highest, respectively, for Black females. The fourth most common cancer site for females is the corpus uteri for both Whites and Blacks. These sites and rates differ from cancers affecting men, where prostate cancer, lung and bronchus, and colon/rectal cancer are most common (USDHHS, 1996). Overall rate for males were 485/100,000 and for women were 344/100,000 in 1991.

Cancer-patient education for women focuses overwhelmingly on breast cancer with much less attention to cervical cancer and even less to the many other malignancies that affect women, female children or adolescents. An encouraging amount of work is being done on effective education for minority women and to a lesser extent older women. Much of the work focuses on assessment of knowledge and beliefs, some on interventions.

MINORITY WOMEN AND CANCER

Many minority groups have greater cancer mortality rates than do Whites and are at the same time less informed about or have less faith in screening procedures and are less likely to participate in them. For example, African Americans as a group have greater colorectal cancer mortality rates, yet are less likely to participate in fecal occult blood testing.

Perceptions of cancer fatalism play a pivotal role in the lack of partici-pation. Cancer fatalism is the belief that death is inevitable when cancer is present. Powe (1995) notes that this belief is no doubt related to the struggles this population has in accessing health care. Her study showed that African Americans had higher cancer fatalism scores that did Cau-casians. These perceptions are more likely to be present among African Americans who are undereducated, have decreased income, and decreased knowledge of colorectal cancer. Unfortunately, strategies for modifying perceptions of cancer fatalism are not yet well articulated.

Although breast cancer incidence is somewhat lower among African American women than among White women in the United States, breast cancer mortality is consistently higher among African Americans in large part because they present with more advanced-stage disease. A number of studies, summarized in Lannin et al. (1998), have shown that there is a large difference among races in breast-cancer knowledge, beliefs, and attitudes, and recent study has shown certain beliefs are associated with late-stage presentation. These include belief that lumps are a normal part of a woman's system and will come and go, and that letting air get to cancer or cutting on it would cause it to spread. Providers should be aware of these beliefs and address them in culturally sensitive ways (Lannin et al., 1998).

Similar findings have been noted with Mexican American women living in southern Texas (Carpenter & Colwell, 1995). A majority of responders had significant misconceptions related to cancer causation, symptoms, and treatment, and expressed feelings of little control over prevention of the disease. Only a minority felt they could undergo the appropriate screenings even if they were available. Only 12% of respon-dents agreed that most cancers can be cured if they are detected early; most (65%) felt they had no control over getting cancer. Fifty-seven percent of the women did not feel comfortable examining their own breasts for lumps. Nearly 40% thought that cancer can be caused by bruises from being hit. About 80% knew breast cancer can be found by breast self-examination (BSE) and mammography and that cancer of the uterus and cervix can easily be found with a Pap smear, 70% knew that eating fruit and vegetables can help prevent colon or rectal cancer. Knowledge and self-efficacy related to performing BSE were highly related as were self-efficacy and cancer screening in general. This sug-gests that improvement of knowledge and other experiences to increase self-efficacy may provide the basis for improving screening and early treatment behaviors.

Latinas may also have culturally based beliefs about cervical cancer that reflect the moral framework within which they interpret disease.

Immigrant Latinas were more likely than U.S.-born Latinas and Anglo women to agree that having multiple sexual partners was a risk factor for cervical cancer. But they were also more likely to believe that poor hygiene, fate, vaginal trauma, abortion, and having sexual intercourse during menses increased the chances of contacting cervical cancer. For breast cancer, these misconceptions included fondling and trauma as increasing the risk. This group was less likely to know the significance of bloody breast discharge and more likely to believe mammograms were necessary only to evaluate lumps (Hubbell, Chavez, Mishra & Valdez, 1996).

The group was also more likely to prefer not to know if they had cervical cancer, to fear telling their spouses, to believe that Pap smears were necessary only in the presence of vaginal bleeding, or that symptoms include bloody stool samples or inguinal rashes. Others reported that Latinas believed cancers were God's punishment for immoral behavior. Indeed, because being given a diagnosis of cervical cancer may imply immoral behavior, one might avoid cancer screening (Hubbell et al., 1996).

In minority populations, low socioeconomic status (SES) may be a barrier to information access and sometimes is also associated with inadequate nutrition. Some also have language barriers and attitudes of fatalism and see suffering as a source of strength. It is important to incorporate culturally sensitive approaches into education of these patients. For example, it can be pointed out that women need not be promiscuous to get cervical cancer. Education is only part of the intervention to support screening behaviors—assessing access to screening services and reminders and other strategies are also important. The presence of all these elements (education, physician encouragement, and reinforcement) have been shown to have the highest yield (Strickland et al., 1997).

OLDER AND POORER WOMEN

Older women are another population with special needs. As a group they are less likely to have mammograms, to be taught BSE, and to have clinical breast examinations than are younger women, particularly if they are women of color, have low educational levels or are poor. Little is known about how proficient elderly women are at performing BSE. Yet, these groups are at highest risk for breast cancer. Because they are frequently isolated, a self-taught educational program including video instruction, printed materials, a miniature lump model, and BSE skill checks raised their proficiency in lump detection (Wood, 1996).

Limited literacy skills and lack of knowledge about screening mammography may contribute considerably to its underutilization in low-income women. Screening for reading level may identify a subset of low-income patients who could benefit from specialized education. Twenty-one percent of adults are functionally illiterate, with 27% possessing marginal literacy skills. These rates are almost twice as high for people living in the inner city and those older than 65 years; yet, these are also the women least likely to get cancer screening. These patients may be unable to comprehend patient education and misunderstand instructions from their physicians. Thirty-nine percent of women reading below a fourth-grade level did not know very basic information that mammography was associated with cancer; many confused it with Pap smears and/or believed that it was not necessary when your breasts looked good or were small. This means that current educational programs and materials are not effective with the most disadvantaged group in society, those with low income and low literacy skills. Screening for low reading level may identify a subset of low-income patients who could benefit from specialized education. Nonprint methods of patient education such as videos, stories, and verbal education by peers are more likely to be successful (Davis et al., 1996).

As with many other fields, the average readability of patient-education materials about prevention, detection, and treatment of breast cancer is about ninth grade, well beyond the reading capability of many women (Glazer, Kirk, & Bosler, 1996). Although knowledge and improving it through education has been discounted by some, a woman's knowledge about proper screening practices does influence screening behavior (Levin et al., 1997).

Examples of educational approaches found to be successful with women from minority populations and older women are included throughout this chapter.

BREAST AND CERVICAL CANCER

After more than two decades of research, only 20%–40% of women in the United States conduct BSE as recommended, and there is little evidence that it is conducted accurately. Research shows that knowledge increases proficiency and accuracy, that information provided through pamphlets and videos needs to be augmented with educational programs and practice, that behavior contracting increases compliance, and that knowledge alone may not be expected to result in the maintenance of doing BSEs as recommended. This combination is congruent with adoption theory, which says that the physician message raises awareness, direct instruction provides knowledge and skills and commitment to do BSE through contracting, and phone and mail contacts provide reinforcement (Strickland et al., 1997).

To add additional reinforcements, others included grocery-store coupons and peer-counseling calls by retired health personnel targeted at older women. Counselors were trained to identify each woman's primary reasons for not scheduling a mammogram and tailored the phone counseling to her concerns. This significantly improved the likelihood of the older women obtaining mammograms. A more intensive intervention may be required for women who have never had a mammogram (Janz et al., 1997).

National data report that Native Americans have one of the highest rates of cervical cancer incidence of any ethnic group studied, and a poorer survival rate. A culturally sensitive program for this group used talking circles to provide cancer education and improve cervical cancer screening. The talking circle is a well-known method of intragroup communication in many Indian communities. The circles involved periodic gathering of 5 to 10 members to share information, support, and problem solving. An arrow, feather, or other talisman was passed around the circle to someone who wished to speak. The Native American tradition is oral and uses stories. Talking circles proved to be an acceptable way to link behavior change to favorable results (Hodge, Fredericks, & Rodriguez, 1996).

Any intervention must build on Native American values of the importance of family, community, cooperation, and harmony with nature. Women in this group may seek native healers for "female" problems and for issues surrounding pregnancy and childbirth (Hodge et al., 1996).

Likewise, the Witness Project managed from the University of Arkansas Health Science Center uses African American cultural traditions to increase awareness and screening for breast cancer in a rural population. Table 5.1 shows how the intervention was designed and implemented and how it used social learning theory. Witnessing occurs in fundamentalist churches in the South when an individual shares with the congregation a personal religious experience. A person witnesses (testifies) by explaining how her/his life has changed through a particular experience.

TABLE 5.1   Social Learning Theory Concepts Applied in the Witness Project™

Environment	Church and local neighborhood-based cueing; social support by role models for questions and problems
Situation	Skills to overcome feelings of helplessness and demonstrate that cancer patients can survive
Behavioral capability	Skills to perform BSE* and resources to obtain Pap tests and mammograms
Expectations	Cancer survivors demonstrate that if you find a cancer early through BSE, mammography, or Pap tests, cancer is not necessarily fatal
Expectancies	"In church, people witness to save souls. In the Witness Project they witness "to save lives." (Witness Project motto)
Observational learning	Direct contact with witness role models for early detection and treatment, as well as other positive health behaviors (nutrition)
Reinforcements	Contact with local witness role models and lay health advisors; providing social reinforcements—i.e. pins, magnets, shower cards, follow-up calls
Self-efficacy	Encourage women to practice BSE, even if they cannot afford mammography; encourage discussion
Reciprocal determination	Promote social support for attention to women's health and the appropriate early detection methods; promote this support through the church, including the pastor and other men

*BSE = breast self-examination.

From Erwin, Deborah O. et al. (1996). Increasing mammography and breast self-examination in African-american women using the Witness Project™ model. *Journal of Cancer Education, 11,* 210–215. Copyright © 1996 by Hanley & Belfus, Inc. Reprinted with permission.

The intended effect of witnessing is to help others who are struggling with serious problems of life, including surviving breast cancer (Erwin et al., 1996).

Again, story telling and experiential learning techniques rather than a traditional didactic presentation are used in the witnessing intervention, because they are more inviting to adults with limited formal education. The Witness Project relied on a team of local African American breast and cervical cancer survivors, "witness role models," who spoke to groups of other African American women at local churches and community organizations. Each talked to the group about her personal experience, highlighting early detection and treatment. The role models challenge excuses women use for not performing BSE or having mammograms. The importance of taking responsibility for one's own health and the need to spread these messages throughout the African American community were emphasized. Participants were taught BSE using ethnic models. Women in the project demonstrated significant increase in the practice of BSE and mammography, although the study lacked a control group. A more detailed explanation may be found in Erwin and colleagues (1996). The authors suggest the Witness Project changes behaviors because the messages are crafted to meet the women's beliefs rather than to change them. The very presence of the witness role models as cancer survivors is evidence supporting God's will.

Distress at a widening racial gap in mammography screening prompted Eng (1993) to use the strength of older rural Black women's social networking to reach those not being screened. "Natural helper" women were trained about cancer to become lay health advisors, to work through their existing kin, friendship, and job networks. They provided social support (especially explanations and referrals) through interpersonal counseling with women in their social networks, and planned and implemented breast cancer control and prevention activities through community-based organizations to which the natural helpers belonged. This approach has a goal not only of reaching target women to assist them to get mammograms but of empowering the community.

These culturally relevant interventions share the common characteristic of honoring culture, local, and religious beliefs rather than changing beliefs to conform to a traditional medical model. These interventions also provide positive experiences to counteract fatalism, negativism, and low knowledge levels, and do not require reading and writing. More traditional interventions have been developed predominantly for educated women. They frequently lack the advocacy and empowerment necessary for special, traditionally underserved populations.

There are demonstrations that what might be thought of as middle-class learning methods will work with impoverished women with low educational levels, if they are properly adapted, however. The Computer Health Enhancement Support System (CHESS) is an interactive computer system containing information, social support, and decision-making and problem-solving tools. It was developed with intensive input from potential users through needs-assessment surveys and field tested with this special population as well as others. All patients dealing with cancer need ready access to these elements, incrementally delivered and easily understood. CHESS modules have been developed for breast cancer and other conditions. Modules include information components (brief answers to common questions, instant library, answers from experts), social support components (discussion groups, personal stories), and problem-solv-

TABLE 5.2   Information Needs of Women After a Breast Biopsy

The types of benign breast
What is fibrocystic disease?

The meaning of risk associated with benign breast disease
What is the meaning of benign breast disease in terms of its risk for developing into breast cancer?
What makes a lump in my breast suspicious for breast cancer?
What are my chances of getting breast cancer?
How long can we wait before having a biopsy and being in real danger of getting breast cancer?

The diagnostic tests required to evaluate a breast lump
How long after my biopsy will I know if my lump is benign or malignant?
How many tests are needed to give a definite diagnosis?
What is involved in the mammographic needle localization procedure?
Do I need follow-up tests or exams if the biopsy is negative?

From Deane, Karen A., & Degner, Lesley F. (1997). Determining the information needs of women after breast biopsy procedures. *AORN Journal, 65,* 767–776. Reprinted by permission.

ing components. Thus CHESS is not only interactive but self-tailored (McTavish et al., 1995).

The educational needs of other groups of women being evaluated for breast cancer are frequently not met. Deane and Degner (1997) describe information needs of a group of women after breast biopsy (see Table 5.2). Participants wanted to understand why a benign breast condition needs to be evaluated and when it represents a risk for development into breast cancer. They were unclear and confused about the purpose of subsequent appointments and other questions. Anxiety levels were found to be three times higher than normal, which can cause poor compliance with early-detection measures. Women with benign results of breast biopsies require education and supportive care and follow-up for their risk factors.

Likewise, long-term survivors of breast cancer live with the ongoing impact of their initial disease experience and continued uncertainty about possible recurrence. Such a group of women reported they could not count on physicians to provide information about: how to monitor their own bodily changes; when and how to take action to have symptoms assessed; how to deal with ongoing effects from treatment for which they had been poorly prepared, especially lymphedema but also fatigue, sexual dysfunction, post treatment menopause and weight gain; how often they should be seen; and how to deal with difficulties in getting or maintaining life or disability insurance. Feelings of abandonment were evident (Gray et al., 1998).

The women had great difficulty in knowing how to access other sources such as pharmacists, nurses, the Internet, telephone information lines, and self-help groups. They also did not understand the confusion and contradictions related to breast cancer treatments and approaches to intervention and were caught in advice that was different from that which they originally received, frequently reflecting changing medical practice. This was particularly the case with tamoxifen (Gray, et al., 1998).

Women continue to be affected by their breast cancer experience many years after treatment ends, even when they have carried on with active, full lives. The ongoing impact of disease is felt strongly around survivors' experience of various aches and pains, in some cases related to posttreatment effects. Uncertain how to interpret physical symptoms, women easily become anxious about the possibilities of a new encounter with cancer. Although it may be that heightened bodily sensitivity is to some degree an unavoidable consequence of cancer experience, it can be less pronounced when cancer survivors are informed about symptoms to be more or less concerned about, and where there are established mechanisms for dealing with them. Too often, breast-cancer survivors are uncertain about when and how to investigate worrisome symptoms. Based on their experiences with physicians and other health professionals, they may become afraid to raise these concerns lest they be seen as neurotic or malingering. It would be an extremely helpful intervention posttreatment to ensure that all patients are provided with guidelines about how to act when they are concerned about physical symptoms (Gray et al., 1998).

Finally, patient education is essential for preparing patients to give informed consent for medical treatment, including screening. In order to consider consenting to, for example, cervical cancer screening, women must have information about: their particular risk of developing cervical cancer, what it will be like to undergo the test (uncomfortable? painful? embarrassing?), potential accuracy of the test including false positives and how often it prevents cancer from developing, and what will happen to them if their smear is positive. Without this knowledge, women may accept an invitation for a smear that then links them into a potentially distressing process of which they are unaware (Foster & Anderson, 1998).

Current medical practice emphasizes the need for health care providers to persuade all women to be screened and frequently does not provide information on the risks and disadvantages to them of being screened. In Great Britain, physicians are provided financial incentives when they reach a targeted proportion of women screened. Foster and Anderson (1998) also note that the exact relationship between high levels of screening and lower mortality rates from cervical cancer is unknown and unproved. It is becoming clear that the number of women diagnosed through screening as having abnormal cells that need treatment is far higher than the number who would go on to develop a life-threatening cancer of the cervix. Supporters of screening programs are convinced that prevention of cervical cancer in a relatively small number of women justifies the possible overtreatment of a larger number of women who have abnormal smear results (Foster & Anderson, 1998).

The authors (Foster & Anderson, 1998) examined patient-education pamphlets distributed to physicians to help them meet screening targets. Many contained material that sounded like propaganda for the test rather than accurate information on women's need for it. Many did not include the items of information listed previously as essential for informed consent. Although screening tests will be seen by many women as beneficial, accurate information and education should be provided to allow them to make their own informed decisions. Incomplete or biased information can undermine women's autonomy, and education that contributes to that can be seen as unethical. This kind of problem need not be limited to cervical cancer screening.

SEEKING CARE

As with other illnesses, noting symptoms and seeking help is also an important focus of education. A meta-analysis of 12 studies estimates that 34% of women with breast-cancer symptoms delay seeking help for 3 or more months. Other work has shown that delay, whether patient or provider, was significantly related to decreased survival. Presenting symptoms other than a lump were associated with significantly greater patient and provider delay. These symptoms include pain, bleeding or discharge, dimpling or tissue thickening, or inverted nipple. Interpreting breast symptoms is more problematic than might be expected. Changes in breast contour were often attributed to clothing constriction, and nipple symptoms were universally treated as skin problems rather than suspected as signs of malignancy (Facione, 1993; Facione & Dodd, 1995). Rather than denying the existence of their breast changes, women reported monitoring their symptom(s) for change.

Clearly, education should include the less common symptoms and need to get to a provider and the limitations of professional breast examination and mammography. Further study with development of research instruments (Facione, Dodd, Holzemer & Meleis, 1997) to test important variables found that prompt help seeking for self-discovered breast-cancer symptoms is dependent on a complex picture of personal, social, and environmental factors. The failure to perceive negative consequences and fatalistic beliefs about developing or dying from breast cancer were strong influences on not seeking help.

The authors suggest that history taking should be expanded to assess women's ideas about: the consequences of delaying evaluation of self-discovered breast symptoms, their sense of vulnerability to breast cancer, the constraints on cancer early detection that they may be feeling related to role obligations, their economic or strategic limitations to accessing such services, and the pressures they might feel to hide a breast cancer symptom. From this assessment, some women may be targeted for education or counseling outreach before the time of symptom occurrence. Help seeking for breast symptoms is not an automatic behavior for all women who need only to be reminded to perform BSE and to follow mammography guidelines (Facione et al, 1997).

Health care systems have frequently not been helpful for women seeking care. If a woman finds a lump in her breast, she often is shuttled between her family physician, a mammography clinic, a surgeon, and a cancer center. Each appointment inevitably involves a delay and lack of communication about what it all means. For such women and their families stress is already very high, and such a nonsystem of care makes it worse. Women's Breast Health Centers, to which women can refer themselves, provide the full range of care in a timely manner, including teaching and assistance with the decisions women need to make (Gray, 1997).

Media messages are a major source of information for many women. Yet, studies of the coverage of breast cancer by popular magazines showed several important inaccuracies. Breast cancer was commonly portrayed as primarily a disease of young, White professional women when it is predominantly a postmenopausal disease with equal African American mortality rates. A common message is that behaviors and choices of young, nontraditional women, especially those related to fertility control, have led to pathological repercussions in their bodies. Mammography, diet, and other changes are said to "prevent" breast cancer, an incorrect statement (Lantz & Booth, 1998).

Colon cancer, the third leading cause of cancer mortality in women, is significantly underreported in comparison to its impact, including in magazines aimed at African American readership. Ovarian and cervical cancers received three times the coverage that colon cancer received in these magazines, yet combined they claimed nearly 100,000 fewer lives than did colon cancer during the years being studied. Few of the articles mentioned age, which is the primary risk factor for this cancer, whereas many mentioned family history although only 5% to 10% of colon cancers have a direct genetic component (Gerlach, Marino, Weed, & Hoffman-Goetz, 1997). Thus media messages can be seriously flawed as educational tools.

HIGH-RISK WOMEN

The concept of being at risk comes from the field of epidemiology and is very influential in national recommendations for changes, including lifestyle changes, that might decrease the chance of developing or contracting a disease. All risks pose problems for the people so diagnosed. One must translate probabilistic statements about populations into terms that have personal meaning even though one has no symptoms, cope with uncertainty, and begin appropriate surveillance and risk reduction. Few studies have examined how individuals understand the risk that has been identified for them. Some studies show that people so identified begin to think of themselves as ill, see their risk as a certainty, and see their bodies as potentially dangerous and liable to destroy them (Kavanagh & Broom, 1998).

Action taken to decrease the risk must occur without any clear confidence in the actual extent of one's personal vulnerability or the ultimate effectiveness of the remedial action. The fact that most diagnoses of risk do not involve symptoms means that the experience of change in symptoms is also not available to judge one's progress in controlling the risk. Many people will be identified for multiple diseases with risk factors that are sometimes genetic. (Kavanagh & Broom, 1998). Interventions that can modify the negative aspects of the risk experience are important.

Of course, patient-education programs frequently incorporate or are built around concepts of risk, and practitioners must struggle with language and approaches that reflect both scientific accuracy and that help people integrate all of this into their lives. Cancer education for women contains many examples of this educational challenge.

Studies of groups of high-risk women highlight the essential nature of good education in positive coping with the risk of breast cancer. Among women with one or more first- degree relatives with breast cancer (and thus at risk twice that of the general female population), as many as half manifested persistent distress related to their risk. Few had their risk assessed in an informed, structured way. All struggled to access, gather, and use information to facilitate adaptation to the threat they faced. When it was available, information preserved hope, promoted adaptation to the relative's cancer illness, encouraged accurate risk perceptions, minimized anxiety, and increased personal control and predictability (Chalmers, Thomson, & Degner, 1996; Chalmers & Luker, 1996). The information was frequently fragmented, inaccurate, inappropriate, or insufficient, and the women felt isolated and frustrated in their attempt to cope with their perceptions of risk. They used personal contacts, the media, and informal written materials. When informational needs are not met, living with the breast cancer experience of their relatives may not be resolved, inaccurate and emotionally devastating risk perception may be developed, and putting risk in its place through cognitive processes and self-care practices may not occur (Chalmers et al., 1996; Chalmers & Luker, 1996).

High-risk women should be identified through mammography clinics, breast cancer treatment centers, and community cancer agencies. Their ability to form an accurate perception and to be confident in self-care to detect breast cancer symptoms should be addressed through individualized information with frequent reinforcement. They must be taken to the level of confidence and competence with tactile BSE and a sense of control over their feelings of risk. This should enable them to carry out regular breast assessments and to act on abnormalities they may find. For many, demonstration alone did not lead to confidence and competence in carrying out BSE, and women who remained unsure seldom pursued this need with their physicians or community resources. Some will find the fear so overwhelming that they don't regularly examine themselves. Information needs and outcomes through the process of becoming an at-risk individual are outlined in Table 5.3. Living the breast-cancer experience refers to the primary relative's illness, which is, of course, a powerful learning experience (Chalmers & Luker, 1996; Chalmers, Thomson, & Degner, 1996).

Women with family histories of breast cancer have a risk of developing the disease that is several times higher than do women in the general population. A group psychoeducational intervention study of women with such family histories (Kash, Holland, Osborne, & Miller, 1995) showed significantly reduced perception of risk (initially at 80% of women overestimating risk by as much as four times greater than their actual risk), and increased adherence to screening behavior. Overestimation of

TABLE 5.3   Information Needs and Outcomes Through the Phases of Becoming an At-Risk Individual

Phase	Information needs	Outcomes
1. Living the breast cancer experience	1. Breast cancer information related to cause and treatment.	1. Preserving hope.
	2. The relative's illness course and prognosis	2. Developing realistic expectations and decreasing uncertainty.
	3. "Normal" physical and emotional responses to breast cancer.	3. Dealing with losses inherent in the cancer illness.
	4. Strategies to alleviate relative's suffering.	4. Finding means of supporting ill relative.
2. Developing risk perception	1. Risk factors associated with breast cancer.	1. Accurate risk perception develop.
	2. Interpretation of personal risk factors to develop a realistic view of risk.	2. Minimizing anxiety.
3. Putting risk in its place	1. Breast cancer detection and prevention strategy.	1. Development of "optimistic worry."
	2. Self-care strategy.	2. Tools to make lifestyle changes.
	3. Monitoring strategy.	3. Sense of self.

From Chalmers, Karen, Thomson, Kathryn, & Degner, Lesley F. (1996). Information, support and communication needs of women with a family history of breast cancer. *Cancer Nursing, 19,* 204–213. Copyright © 1996 by Lippincott, Williams & Wilkins. Reproduced with permission.

risk can be a major barrier to screening. The higher a woman's perception of risk the less she adheres to regular mammograms and clinical breast exams (CBEs) and the less she performs monthly BSE because she fears finding a lump.

Women who are at risk of developing breast cancer because of their strong family histories are also at higher risk for psychological distress. These women frequently describe themselves as "walking time bombs," 100% sure they will get breast cancer. Those who feel they have passed a gene to their daughters or who have not yet developed breast cancer while other relatives have feel "survivor" guilt. They feel helpless toward the disease and experience a lack of self-efficacy regarding its prevention. The intervention provided these women with objective risk status, information and development of self-efficacy on ways to take control of their lifestyle, emotional support and clarification of information about breast cancer and risk factors. They were then able to estimate their risk accurately, increased their knowledge of breast cancer and improved adherence to screening behaviors. The women in the control group (who were provided only risk counseling) continued to increase their perception of risk over time. Booster sessions were needed.

The availability of genetic testing for BRCa mutations creates its own need for careful education. Tessaro, Borstelmann, Regan, Rimer, and Winer (1997) found a general lack of very basic knowledge about genetic testing for breast cancer, particularly what it would mean to have a positive test result. Several confused it with screening for breast cancer. A lack of proven options after testing was a major concern, as was confidentiality of information and possible loss of insurance coverage. Women needed information about genetic counseling before receiving it. Only a third considered themselves adequately prepared, which they believed kept them from obtaining a definitive risk estimate. Suggested content for a leaflet developed for this purpose may be found in Table 5.4 (Hallowell, Murton, Statham, Green, & Richards, 1997). Because of

TABLE 5.4 Suggested Content of Information Leaflet About Genetic Counseling

Description of process of genetic counseling as practiced in clinic—This should inform counsellees about what will occur during their consultation: that their family health history will be discussed, whether blood may be taken, and whether screening or physical examination may be performed. It should also emphasize that counselling is a two-way exchange and encourage counsellees to prepare questions for the counsellor. An indication of whether it would be appropriate for a partner or close relative to attend the consultation would be helpful

Description of content of genetic discussions—This should outline the topics that may be discussed during the consultation: family history, risk assessment, and options for risk management for both counsellee and relatives. A list of all the details of the family history that the counsellee needs to bring to the consultation should be included. It should be emphasized that information about all known blood relatives, male and female and not just those affected by cancer, may be helpful

Background information—This should include brief epidemiological facts about the cancers (for example, the population risk of breast cancer is 1 in 12 and about 5% of cases of breast cancer are caused by an inherited predisposition), a simplified illustration of autosomal dominant inheritance, and a brief description of current research into cancer genes and the implications for DNA testing

This table was first published in the BMJ [Hallowell, N., Munton, F., Statham, H., Green, J. M., & Richards, M. P. M. (1997). Women's need for information before attending genetic counseling for familial breast or ovarian cancer: A questionnaire, interview and observational study. *British Medical Journal, 314:* 281–283] and is reproduced by permission of the BMJ.

the psychological and social risks to patients of being identified as susceptible to a genetic disorder, it is important that education take place
before a patient undergoes genetic testing.

Access to education about genetic susceptiblity to breast cancer is
problematic. Many primary care providers have limited knowledge, time,
and confidence with the subject matter, and genetic counselors are not
widely available to all who might need education and counseling. A CD-
ROM is available to provide the information outlined in Table 5.4, with
interactive questions to assure patient learning. Visuals show how much
gene mutation status affects the risk of developing breast cancer. Future
versions will include videotaped interviews of actual patients describing
their experiences. Whether such a method can replace one-on-one counseling methods remains to be seen, but it clearly can provide an educational base for counseling (Green & Fost, 1997).

TEACHING TOOLS AND APPROACHES

General teaching approaches are thoroughly described in general patient-education sources (Redman, 1997). Several examples specific to
cancer in women are described here.

The Internet contains a number of sources of information for patients
and families to access. The National Cancer Institute maintains a site
called Breast Cancer for Patients, which includes information on treatment, quality of life, diagnosis, prevention, risk factors, and genetics.
The American Cancer Society's Illustrated Guide to Breast Self-Efficacy
is available on Oncolink. Other available information includes treatment
for advanced breast cancer, unconventional therapies, clinical trials, breast
reconstruction, how to deal with lymphedema, support groups and advocacy (Pillar, 1997).

Incorporation of sensory information into teaching about procedures
to be used in cancer diagnosis or care in women offer the opportunity
for more positive coping. Nugent and Clark (1996) describe the development of sensory information for colposcopy (a diagnostic procedure
used to determine if cancer is present in the cervix whan a Pap examination shows cervical changes). Women who have just completed the
procedure are interviewed about the sensations they experienced during
it—what they noticed, heard, saw, smelled, or tasted. A sufficient num-

TABLE 5.5   Sensory Information Message for Colposcopy

Once you have changed into a hospital gown for the procedure, you will be taken to the colposcopy room. In the room, you will notice an examining table with stirrups, a cart holding instruments, and the colposcope (a piece of equipment that looks like a microscope). You will be asked to get up on the examining table and to slide down on the table so that your feet are in the stirrups. A clinician will explain the procedure to you either before it is done or as it is being done.

The clinician may perform a pelvic examination. Then, he/she inserts a speculum, which will feel cool and uncomfortable. Once the speculum is in place, the clinician will clean and examine your cervix. He/she also will apply vinegar to your cervix. The vinegar helps the clinical to see any abnormal area(s) better. The vinegar will feel cool.

The clinician may take a sample of secretions from your cervical canal. This means that he/she would quickly move a probe in and out of the cervix. If this is part of your examination you will feel a cramping sensation that will last as long as it takes to obtain the sample.

The clinician will take a biopsy specimen of any abnormal area(s) on the cervix. You will likely hear a snipping sound as the clamps come together and feel a pinch as the biopsy is being taken. The pinching sensation lasts only seconds.

The clinician will remove the speculum, which will give you a sense of relief. It may seem as though the speculum is being removed more slowly than it is when you have a Pap test. The reason for the difference is that the clinician can use the colposcope to take a good look at the top part of your vagina.

The clinician may also examine your external genitals. If this is part of your examination, he/she will spray vinegar on this area so that any abnormal area(s) are seen more easily. The vinegar will feel cool.

The procedure is now completed. You are asked to sit up on the side of the examining table. You will be given information about how and when you will receive the biopsy result.

From Nugent, L. S., & Clark, C. R. (1996). Colposcopy: Sensory information for client education. *Journal of Obstetric, Gynecologic, & Neonatal Nursing, 25,* 225–231. Copyright © Lippincott, Williams & Wilkins. Reprinted with permission.

ber are interviewed to determine their degree of agreement. The message so developed for colposcopy appears as Table 5.5.

McDaniel and Rhodes (1998) developed a preparatory sensory information videotape for women receiving chemotherapy for breast cancer. The information, which varied by protocol, included experiences before, during, and after chemotherapy, as experienced by the women undergoing them. Metallic taste, increased sensitivity to odors, changes in temperature with administration, itching, blurring vision, feeling woozy or faint were included. Preparatory sensory information is not usually included in standard chemotherapy care yet has been shown to be highly efficacious for other procedures. Relaxation and imagery may also be used.

MEASUREMENT INSTRUMENTS

Increasingly, patient-education practice uses validated measurement tools for purposes of patient assessment and evaluation of the effectiveness of interventions. Several such tools specific to the care of women or that have been considerably used with women, are included here. Others that could be used in oncology practice are included in Redman (1998). Assessment of information needs of women with recent diagnosis of breast cancer can be accomplished using the Toronto Informational Needs Questionnaire—Breast Cancer (TINQ-BC), developed by Galloway and others (1997). A copy, description, and critique of this instrument may be found in a compilation of patient-education measurement tools (Redman, 1998). Subscales focus on measurement of information needs about the disease, diagnostic procedures, treatments, physician, and psychosocial needs. Patients frequently show high need for information (Galloway et al., 1997).

Dibble, Padilla, Dodd, and Miaskowski (1998) show that measurement of quality of life for cancer requires gender-specific questions to accurately address the dimensions of this concept in males and females. Results of a factor analysis of the Multidimensional Quality of Life Scale—Cancer Version (MQOLS-CA) (now known as the Quality of Life Scale), showed that women and men can perceive the same items differently and that items cluster together in different ways for each gender. The revised Quality of Life instrument contains 10 items similar for both genders and additional unique items for men and women.

The authors suggest a broader implication for measurement. Rather than report normative data for instruments that suggest women are more anxious, more depressed, and have more negative mood states than do men, separate factor-analytic procedures (nonconfirmatory) should be performed by gender to establish if the essential components of these emotions are gender specific. This procedure is perhaps especially important for quality-of-life measurement as this construct is rapidly becoming one of the outcomes for clinical trials. Studies identifying gender-specific antecedents would then provide information for targeted interventions to be developed and tested to affect quality of life directly or through impact of the intervention on a specific antecedent (Dibble et al., 1998).

Breast Cancer Knowledge Test

Developed by Jennifer Lou Stager

Because studies in some patient populations have found that increasing women's knowledge about breast carcinoma risks and screening benefits favorably influences their screening behavior, an instrument by which to assess this knowledge should be useful (Dolan, Lee, & McDermott, 1997). The Breast Cancer Knowledge Test (BCKT), found in Table 5.6, assesses screening and detection knowledge. Content valdity was supported by four oncology experts. In testing with 182 women, 91% Anglo American, internal consistency was .60 for the General Knowledge subscale and .62 for the Curability subscale, with an overall alpha of .71. An additional scale measures knowledge about detection and screening practices (labeled Posttested BCK Test) (McCance, Mooney, Smith & Field, 1990). Testing with 101 women older than 50 years showed internal consistency reliability of .81. Completing all three scales takes about 10 minutes (Stager, 1993).

Use of an adaptation of this tool showed understanding that prevalence of breast cancer increases with age. It also documented that older women were more likely to believe myths including the false notion that once a lump is detected, it is too late to treat it effectively (Dolan et al., et., 1997). It must be noted that the relationship between knowledge and frequency of practice of BSE and mammography is inconsistent (McCance et al., 1990; Stager, 1993).

Another instrument focusing on measurement of knowledge about breast cancer may be found in Vaeth (1993). It assesses knowledge about breast-cancer treatment, misconceptions, risks, and symptoms and is psychometrically in early stages of development.

TABLE 5.6   Breast Cancer Knowledge Test

General knowledge

1. A hard blow to the breast may cause a woman to get breast cancer later in life. (FALSE)
2. The constant irritation of a tight bra can, over time, cause breast cancer. (FALSE)
3. One out of every 10 women in the United States will get breast cancer some time during her life. (TRUE).
4. In some women, being overweight increases the risk of developing breast cancer. (TRUE)
5. A woman who bears her first child before the age of 30 is more likely to develop breast cancer than a woman who bears her first child after the age of 30. (FALSE)
6. Women with no known risk factors for breast cancer rarely get breast cancer. (FALSE)
7. Some types of fibrocystic breast disease (noncancerous breast lumps) increase a woman's risk of breast cancer. (TRUE)
8. Women in the United States have a higher risk of breast cancer than do women in Asia or Africa. (TRUE)
9. Breast cancer is more common in 65–year-old women than in 40–year-old women. (TRUE)
10. The most frequently occurring cancer in women is breast cancer. (TRUE)
11. Women over age 70 rarely get breast cancer. (FALSE)
12. Most breast lumps are cancerous. (FALSE)

Curability

1. For many women, breast cancer can now be successfully treated without breast removal (mastectomy). (TRUE)
2. By the time a cancerous breast lump is painful, it is too late to be successfully treated. (FALSE)
3. If all lymph glands around the breast and under the arm are not removed, breast cancer cannot be cured. (FALSE)
4. Breast cancer is sometimes treated successfully by removal of the lump (lumpectomy) and radiation therapy. (TRUE)
5. Breast cancer is less likely to be cured in women with a family history of breast cancer than in women with no family history of breast cancer. (FALSE)
6. By the time a woman can feel a cancerous breast lump, it is too late to treat it effectively. (FALSE)
7. Even if breast cancer is caught very early, the chances for cure are much better if the whole breast is removed. (FALSE)
8. Even if detected and treated early, a woman with breast cancer is unlikely to live a normal life span. (FALSE)

*At the time of testing statistics indicated that one woman in ten in the United States will get breast cancer sometime in her life. Currently that figure is one in nine.

From Stager, Jennifer Lou. (1993). The comprehensive breast cancer knowledge test: Validity and reliability. *Journal of Advanced Nursing, 18,* 1133–1140. Copyright © 1993 Blackwell Science Ltd. Reprinted by permission.

Beliefs About Mammography and Breast Self-Examination (Also Known As Champion's Health Belief Scale)

Developed by Victoria Champion and Catherine R. Scott

This tool is based on the Health Belief Model (HBM), a cognitive, attitudinal model that has been broadly applied across disease entities and areas of health prevention. This specific tool posits that breast-cancer screening behaviors are the result of decision making based on: (a) perceived susceptibility to breast cancer, (b) perceived seriousness of breast cancer, (c) perceived benefits of screening actions, (d) perceived barriers to screening actions, and (e) self-efficacy to accomplish screening actions. Perceived susceptibility and seriousness are related to the individual's knowledge of the disease and personal risk factors, which may or not be accurate. Higher personal perception of susceptibility to breast cancer has been reported as being significantly related to breast-cancer screening behavior. A problem associated with perceived seriousness as a predictor has been lack of variability in responses; almost all women perceive breast cancer as extremely serious (Champion & Miller, 1992).

From this model, perceived benefits and barriers have been found to be predictive of mammography. Women who perceive many barriers to mammography are more likely to be noncompliant; those with positive beliefs are more likely to have mammography (Champion, 1995). Therefore, measurement of benefits and barriers constructs is important. Although both have been consistently related to BSE, barriers have accounted for the most variance in BSE behavior (Champion, 1993). For mammography and provider breast exam (PBE), susceptibility, social influence, and knowledge related to it were important. Complete breast cancer screening requires that BSE, mammography, and PBE be completed routinely (Champion, 1991).

The Breast Cancer Screening Belief Scales may be seen in Table 5.7. Responses range from strongly agree (5) to strongly disagree (1). Content validity was established through consensus of national experts including those expert with HBM constructs. Internal consistency reliability coefficients ranged from .73–.79 for mammography benefits and barriers scales, respectively, to .80 and .88 for BSE benefits and barriers scales. Perceived susceptibility had an internal consistency reliability coefficient of .93 and confidence for BSE at .88. Test–retest reliabilities range from .40–.68 with the BSE mammography and benefits scales. The instrument is at the fifth-grade reading level.

TABLE 5.7   Breast Cancer Screening Belief Scales

Susceptibility

"It is extremely likely that I will get breast cancer."

"My chances of getting breast cancer ill the next few years are great."

"I feel I will get breast cancer sometime during my life.""

"Developing breast cancer is currently a possibility for me."

"I am concerned about the likelihood of developing breast cancer in the near future."

Benefit mammography

"Having a mammogram will help me find breast lumps early."

"If I find a lump early through a mammogram my treatment for breast cancer may not be as bad."

"Having a mammogram is the best way for me to find a very small breast lump."

"Having a mammogram will decrease my chances of dying from breast cancer."

Benefit BSE

"When I do BSE I am doing something to take care of myself."

"Completing BSE each month may help me to find breast lumps early."

"Completing BSE each month may decrease my chances of dying from breast cancer."

"If I find a lump early through BSE, my treatment for breast cancer may not be as bad."

Barrier mammography

"I am afraid to find out there is something wrong when I have a mammogram."

"I am afraid to have a mammogram because I don't understand what will be done."

"I don't know how to go about scheduling a mammogram."

"Having a mammogram would be embarrassing."

"Having a mammogram would take too much time."

"Having a mammogram would be painful."

"People doing the mammogram are nice to women."

"Having a mammogram would expose me to unnecessary radiation."

"It is difficult to get transportation for a mammogram."

"It is difficult to get child care to get a mammogram."

"I have other problems more important than getting a mammogram."

"Having a mammogram costs too much money."

"I cannot remember to schedule an appointment for a mammogram."

Barrier BSE

"I do not feel I can do breast examination correctly."

"Doing BSE will make me worry about what is wrong with my breast."

"BSE is embarrassing to me."

"BSE takes too much time."

"It is hard to remember to do breast examination."

"I don't have enough privacy to do breast examination."

"BSE is not necessary if you have a breast exam by a health care provider."

"BSE is not necessary if you have a routine mammogram."

"My breasts are too large for me to complete breast self-examination."

"My breasts are too lumpy for me to complete breast examination."

"I have other problems more important than doing breast self-examination."

(continued)

TABLE 5.7 (Continued)

BSE self-efficacy
  "I know how to perform BSE."
  "I can perform BSE correctly."
  "I could find a breast lump by performing BSE."
  "I am able to find a breast lump which is the size of a quarter."
  "I am able to find a breast lump which is the size of a dime."
  "I am able to find a breast lump which is the size of a pea."
  "I am sure of the steps to follow for doing BSE."
  "I am able to tell something is wrong with my breasts when doing breast self-examination."
  "I am able to tell something is wrong with my breasts when I look in the mirror."
  "I can use the correct part of my fingers when examining my breasts."

Note. BSE = breast self-examination.

From Champion, Victoria L., & Scott, Catherine R. (1997). Reliability and validity of breast cancer screening belief scales in African-American women. *Nursing Research, 46,* 331–337. Copyright © Lippincott, Williams & Wilkins. Reprinted with permission.

The measurement characteristics of these scales have now been studied with multiple populations with stable results. Factor analysis supports the unidimensionality of both the benefits and the barriers scales. Low correlations with outcome behaviors indicate that the scales require more work, especially with older women, and to determine which items are more relevant for predicting mammogram use. Also important is study of the scales relative to the stages of adopting behaviors outlined in the transtheoretical model.

Focus groups among low-income African American women provided imput for revision. Specific items addressing barriers relevant to this population were added. Barriers more relevant to this population than to a White middle-class population include: lack of understanding about the mammogram procedure and scheduling it, child care and transportation, and rude health care providers. Consistent with results from other populations are barriers of worry, embarrassment, time, pain, and money. Results from factor analysis support validity of this tool, and theoretically specified relationships between the scales and cancer-screening behaviors showing low correlations in the expected direction. The authors (Champion & Scott, 1997) believe that the revised scales have acceptable reliability and validity for this population; low test–retest reliability may be explained by actual changes in beliefs between testing.

The scales have also been used to study the beliefs of rural Appalachian women, whose culture is self-contained, family oriented with a strong set of fundamentalist religious values, and present oriented. Their mean scores and standard deviations for the scales were: confidence

37.9 (9.7); health motivation 27.7 (4.4); susceptibility 13.8 (4.9); seriousness 23.7 (5.5); benefits 22.7 (4.7); and barriers 12.8 (5.4). Only two of the scales (confidence, benefits) were significantly related to reports of doing BSE (Sortet & Banks, 1997).

A theoretically driven intervention study (Champion, 1994) showed that women receiving teaching tailored to their own beliefs about susceptibility, barriers, and benefits and information about mammography were five times more likely than those in the control group to comply with mammography recommendations in the following year. Significant changes in all beliefs except susceptibility occurred following intervention, and the scales were shown to be sensitive to intervention. Other studies have consistently found physician recommendations to be very important (Aiken, West, Woodward, & Reno, 1994)

HEALTH POLICY

It is important to understand how the good that education can do is profoundly influenced by health policies. For example, it is national policy in Great Britain that women over 65 years of age are not invited to receive breast cancer screening but can be screened on request. Few older women are aware of their rising risk of breast cancer with age, or of the value and availability of screening. Those who try to refer themselves face barriers, and fewer than 2% of the eligible population are screened. This occurs even though studies indicate that screening 65–69-year-olds confers benefits similar to those seen in 50–64-year-olds: a 25% decrease in breast cancer mortality. The press regularly carries stories of breast cancer in young women, ignoring the predominance of the disease in older women. This policy has properly been labelled as ageist, indicating a stereotyped negative view of older people that leads to policy decisions that disadvantage them (Sutton, 1997).

Through the efforts of activists, Breast Cancer Informed Consent laws were passed in 18 states during the 1980s. These laws require, variously, that treatment information on alternatives to radical mastectomy be given to patients, that consent be obtained from the patient prior to surgery, and that there be a penalty for physician noncompliance (Anglin, 1997).

SUMMARY

The experience of cancer provides several lessons in education for women. (a) When they have health concerns, some women turn to other women with similar experiences for social support and information. (b) Culturally relevant approaches can be developed and used. (c) Interpreting symptoms is more problematic than might be expected. Thus, judgments of ignorance or lack of knowledge on the part of those who delay may be unfair and ignore realities of the somatic experiences. (d) Knowledge, access to care, and self-efficacy about self-care are important predictors of women's managing their cancer risk (Champion & Menon, 1997). (e) Policies for access to services limit or enhance the effectiveness education can have. There are strong contemporary examples of policy bias and of activism to address policy issues believed not to be supportive of the well-being of women.

REFERENCES

Aiken, L. S., West, S. G., Woodward, C. K., & Reno, R. R. (1994). Health beliefs and compliance with mammography-screening recommendations in asymptomatic women. *Health Psychology, 13,* 122–129.

Anglin, M. K. (1997). Working from the inside out: Implications of breast cancer activism for biomedical policies and practices. *Social Science & Medicine, 44,* 1403–1415.

Carpenter, V., & Colwell, B. (1995). Cancer knowledge, self-efficacy, and cancer screening behaviors among Mexican-American women. *Journal of Cancer Education, 10,* 217–222.

Chalmers, K. I., & Luker, K. A. (1996). Breast self-care practices in women with primary relatives with breast cancer. *Journal of Advanced Nursing, 23,* 1212–1220.

Chalmers, K., Thomson, K., & Degner, L. F. (1996). Information, support, and communication needs of women with a family history of breast cancer. *Cancer Nursing, 19,* 204–213.

Champion, V. L. (1991). The relationship of selected variables to breast cancer detection behaviors in women 35 and older. *Oncology Nursing Forum, 18,* 733–739.

Champion, V. L. (1993). Instrument refinement for breast cancer screening behaviors. *Nursing Research, 42,* 139–143.

Champion, V. L. (1994). Strategies to increase mammography utilization. *Medical Care, 32,* 118–129.

Champion, V. (1995). Development of a benefits and barriers scale for mammography utilization. *Cancer Nursing, 18,* 53–59.

Champion, V., & Menon, U. (1997). Predicting mammography and breast self-examination in African American women. *Cancer Nursing, 20,* 315–322.

Champion, V. L., & Miller, T. K. (1992). Variables related to breast self-examination. *Psychology of Women Quarterly, 16,* 81–96.

Champion, V. L., & Scott, C. R. (1997). Reliability and validity of breast cancer screening belief scales in African American women. *Nursing Research, 46,* 331–337.

Davis, T. C., Arnold, C., Berkel, H. J., Nandy, I., Jackson, R. H., & Glass, J. (1996). Knowledge and attitude on screening mammography among low-literate, low-income women. *Cancer, 78,* 1912–1920.

Deane, K. A., & Degner, L. F. (1997). Determining the information needs of women after breast biopsy procedures. *Association of Operating Room Nurses Journal, 65,* 767–776.

Dibble, S. L., Padilla, G. V., Dodd, M. J., & Miaskowski, C. (1998). Gender differences in the dimensions of quality of life. *Oncology Nursing Forum, 25,* 577–583.

Dolan, N. C., Lee, A. M., & McDermott, M. M. (1997). Age-related differences in breast carcinoma knowledge, beliefs, and perceived risk among women visiting an academic general medical practice. *Cancer, 80,* 413–420.

Eng, E. (1993). The Save Our Sisters Project. *Cancer, 72,* 1071–1077.

Erwin, D. O., Spatz., T. S., Ches, R., Stotts, C., Hollenberg, J. A., & Deloney, L. A. (1996). Increasing mammography and breast self-examination in African American women using the Witness Project model. *Journal of Cancer Education, 11,* 210–215.

Facione, N. C. (1993). Delay versus help seeking for breast cancer symptoms: A critical review of the literature on patient and provider delay. *Social Science & Medicine, 12,* 1521–1534.

Facione, N. C., & Dodd, M. J. (1995). Women's narratives of helpseeking for breast cancer. *Cancer Practice, 3,* 219–225.

Facione, N. C., Dodd, M. J., Holzemer, W., & Meleis, A. I. (1997). Helpseeking for self-discovered breast symptoms. *Cancer Practice, 5,* 220–227.

Foster, P., & Anderson, C. M. (1998). Reaching targets in the national cervical screening programme: Are current practices unethical? *Journal of Medical Ethics, 24,* 151–157.

Galloway, S., Graydon, J., Harrison, D., Evans-Boyden, B., Palmer-Wickham, S., Burlein-Hall, S., Rich-van der Bij, L., West, P., & Blair, A. (1997). Informational needs of women with a recent diagnosis of breast cancer:

Development and initial testing of a tool. *Journal of Advanced Nursing* 25, 1175–1183.

Gerlach, K. K., Marino, C., Weed, D. L., & Hoffman-Goetz, L. (1997). Lack of colon cancer coverage in seven women's magazines. *Women & Health, 26,* 57–68.

Glazer, H. R., Kirk, L. M., & Bosler, F. E. (1996). Patient education pamphlets about prevention, detection, & treatment of breast cancer for low literacy women. *Patient Education & Counseling, 27,* 185–189.

Gray, C. (1997). One-stop care at breast centre another sign of patients' increasing influence. *Canadian Medical Association Journal, 157,* 1419–1420.

Gray, R. E., Fitch, M., Greenberg, M., Hampson, A., Doherty, M., & Labrecque, M. (1998). The information needs of well, longer-term survivors of breast cancer. *Patient Education & Counseling, 33,* 245–255.

Green, M. J., & Fost, N. (1997). An interactive computer program for educating and counseling patients about genetic susceptibility to breast cancer. *Journal of Cancer Education, 12,* 204–208.

Hallowell, N., Murton, F., Statham, H., Green, J. M., & Richards, M. P. M. (1997). Women's need for information before attending genetic counselling for familial breast or ovarian cancer: A questionnaire, interview, and observational study. *British Medical Journal, 314,* 281–283.

Hodge, F., Fredericks, L., & Rodriguez, B. (1996). American Indian women's talking circle. *Cancer, 78,* 1592–1592.

Hubbell, F. A., Chavez, L. R., Mishra, S. I., & Valdez, R. B. (1996). Beliefs about sexual behavior and other predicators of Papanicolau smear screening among Latinas and Anglo women. *Archives of Internal Medicine, 156,* 2353–2358.

Janz, N. K., Schottenfeld, D., Doerr, K. M., Selig, S. M., Dunn, R. L., Strawderman, M., & Levine, P. A. (1997). A two-step intervention to increase mammography among women aged 65 & older. *American Journal of Public Health, 87,* 1683–1686.

Kash, K. M., Holland, J. C., Osborne, M. P., & Miller, D. G. (1995). Psychological counseling strategies for women at risk of breast cancer. *Journal of the National Cancer Institute Monographs, 17,* 73–79.

Kavanagh, A. M., & Broom, D. H. (1998). Embodied risk: My body, myself? *Social Science & Medicine, 46,* 437–444.

Lannin, D. R., Mathews, H. F., Mitchell, J., Swanson, M. S., Swanson, F. H., & Edwards, M. S. (1998). Influence of socioeconomic and cultural factors on racial differences in late-stage presentation of breast cancer. *Journal of the American Medical Association, 279,* 1801–1807.

Lantz, P. M., & Booth, K. M. (1998). The social construction of the breast cancer epidemic. *Social Science & Medicine, 46,* 907–918.

Levin, J. R., Hirsch, S., Bastani, R., Ganz, P. A., Lovett, M. L., & Reuben, D.

B. (1997). Acceptability of mobile mammography among community-dwelling older women. *Journal of the American Geriatrics Society, 45,* 1365–1370.

McCance, K. L., Mooney, K. H., Smith, K. R., & Field, R. (1990). Validity & reliability of a breast cancer knowledge test. *American Journal of Preventive Medicine, 6,* 93–98.

McDaniel, R. W., & Rhodes, V. A. (1998). Development of a preparatory sensory information videotape for women receiving chemotherapy for breast cancer. *Cancer Nursing, 21,* 143–148.

McTavish, F. M., Gustafson, D. H., Owens, B. H., Hawkins, R. P., Pingree, S., Wise, M., Taylor, J. O., & Apantaku, F. M. (1995). CHESS: An interactive computer system for women with breast cancer piloted with an underserved population. *Journal of Ambulatory Care Management, 18,* 35–41.

Nugent, L. S., & Clark, C. R. (1996). Colposcopy: Sensory information for client information. *Journal of Obstetric, Gynecologic, and Neonatal Nursing, 25,* 225–231.

Pillar, C. (1997). Breast cancer information on the Internet. *Health Care on the Internet, 1,* 57–65.

Powe, B. D. (1995). Perceptions of cancer fatalism among African Americans: The influence of education, income, and cancer knowledge. *Journal of the National Black Nurses Association, 7(2),* 41–48.

Redman, B. K. (1997). *The practice of patient education* (8th ed.). St. Louis: Mosby.

Redman, B. K. (1998). *Measurement tools in patient education.* New York: Springer Publishing Co.

Sortet, J. P., & Banks, S. R. (1997). Health beliefs of rural Appalachian women & the practice of breast self-examination. *Cancer Nursing, 20,* 231–235.

Stager, J. L. (1993). The comprehensive Breast Cancer Knowledge Test: Validity & reliability. *Journal of Advanced Nursing, 18,* 1133–1140.

Strickland, C. J., Feigl, P., Upchurch, C., King, D. K., Pierce, H. I., Grevtad, P. K., Bearden, J. D., Dawson, M., Loewen, W. C., & Mayskens, F. L. (1997). Improving breast self-examination compliance: A Southwest Oncology Group randomized trial of three interventions. *Preventive Medicine, 26,* 320–332.

Sutton, G. C. (1997). Will you still need me, will you still screen me, when I'm past 64? *British Medical Journal, 315,* 1032–1033.

Tessaro, I., Borstelmann, N., Regan, K., Rimer, B. K., & Winer, E. (1997). Genetic testing for susceptibility to breast cancer: Findings from women's focus groups. *Journal of Women's Health, 6,* 317–327.

Vaeth, P. A. (1993). Women's knowledge about breast cancer. *American Journal of Clinical Oncology, 16,* 446–454.

U. S. Department of Health and Human Services, National Institutes of Health,

National Cancer Institute (1996). *Cancer rates and risks* (4th ed.). Washington, DC: U.S. Government Printing office.

Wood, R. Y. (1996). Breast self-examination proficiency in older women: Measuring the efficacy of video self-instruction kits. *Cancer Nursing, 19,* 420–436.

CHAPTER SIX

AIDS and Sexually Transmitted Disease Education

T he Centers for Disease Control and Prevention (1997) has gathered statistics from states with confidential HIV infection reporting and determined that at the end of 1997, 23,887 women and 68,210 men were HIV infected but had not yet developed AIDS. At that same time, the number of reported cases of AIDS was 102,383 women affected and 538,703 men. No doubt others remain unreported.

The number of AIDS cases among U. S. women has been rising steadily and has increased more in women than men in recent years largely because of the increase in women infected through heterosexual contact. Half of the cases are the result of intravenous drug use and another 20% from sexual contact with men who are intravenous drug users (IDUs). Black women die from AIDS at many times the rate of White women (O'Leary, Jemmott, Goodhart, & Gebelt, 1996). There is a larger pool of infected men and women run a greater risk than do heterosexual men, of encountering an HIV-infected sexual partner. Transmission is many times more efficient from male to female than the reverse.

AIDS education for women presents a classic case of the politics of class, gender, and race. Interventions to prevent HIV infection in women and infants have largely been aimed at getting women to persuade their partners to use condoms and avoiding sex with high-risk partners (Galavotti et al., 1995).

The backdrop to all of this is the delayed recognition by the medical community of HIV symptoms specific to women. The first natural-history study of HIV disease in women commenced in 1992 about the same time that the Centers for Disease Control and Prevention first recognized that HIV symptoms specific to women existed. These actions occurred 10 years after AIDS was first reported in women. The result was that many women didn't get the care they needed (Cooper, 1995).

Lack of testing of drugs in women meant that the scientific base for treatment was insufficient. Lack of availability of drug-treatment programs for women who were pregnant or HIV-positive added to their difficulty in getting treatment for a major way of contracting HIV. For HIV positive pregnant women, the focus was on their infants and not on the health of the mothers. Espousal by some of a policy of mandatory testing implicitly assumed that women could not be trusted to make good decisions for themselves and their infants. When HIV-related counseling was offered universally in prenatal and delivery settings and testing was voluntary, confidential, and linked to available care and services, 90% of pregnant women consented to testing (Cooper, 1995). In addition, focus has been on the impact of a positive antibody test on women's childbearing decisions with little attention to childbearing decisions of HIV-positive men.

HIV AND AIDS EDUCATION AMONG VARIOUS GROUPS OF WOMEN

African American and Latino women as groups are at particularly high risk of becoming HIV infected. Latino women have the additional concern that condom use is against the official policy of the Roman Catholic church. The African American community has had concerns about genocide related to the HIV epidemic. In addition, women at highest risk already face a multitude of other problems including poverty, substance abuse, alcoholism, violence, unemployment, and unplanned pregnancy (Wortley & Fleming, 1997).

Because risk-reduction strategies have focused on use of male condoms, women cannot control their use and must negotiate it with their partners. For some women, this negotiation may lead to physical harm or financial abandonment as well as serious disruption of relationships. Policies that place responsibility for condom use on women and use education to convince them that this is their responsibility are unfair. The ideology of individual responsibility bolsters the fiction that all members of society are equally capable of controlling the social circumstances that affect their health. Knowledge of HIV transmission and its prevention does little good if women do not have the necessary social status and economic independence to negotiate sexual relations with their partners. Lack of self-esteem also increases vulnerability (O'Leary et al., 1996).

Because condom negotiation and social skills that women must learn are complex and developing motivation is essential, education must be of high intensity and individualized to assure that the skills are gained. This negotiation is often done in the face of numerous partner objections. Condom requests can be taken as suggesting partner unfaithfulness, the possibility of disease, and disregard for his sexual pleasure. The most successful interventions are behavioral, using cognitive social theory, and emphasizing observation, modeling, self-efficacy beliefs and social reinforcement for sustaining behavioral changes. They are also peer led and address gender relations. Multiple sessions provide information to increase awareness and knowledge of risks associated with specific practices, development of social and self-management skills and a sense of self-efficacy in using them in a variety of social situations, and creation of social support (Wingood & DiClemente, 1996).

Men should be targeted for education directly rather than through women. There is evidence that the behaviors they must learn (using condoms) are less complex and therefore that low-intensity interventions that do not need to create individualized skill building will be effective. In some populations of males, information, motivation enhancement, and condom availability may be enough to produce behavior change (O'Leary et al., 1996).

A group with almost no educational resources is lesbian women. It is now believed that woman-to-woman transmission is possible although no precise rates are known. HIV has been detected in cervical and vaginal secretions throughout the menstrual cycle. Concurrent STD, especially ulcerative conditions; sores on the lips and mouth; and transfer of fluids by hand, glove or toy provide a transmission route (White, 1997). Lesbian and bisexual women are among the least studied, least understood of the populations affected by AIDS. This means they have not had access to resources including education, which they need to understand their risk and how to adequately protect themselves. A large study of this population (Stevens, 1994) found many did not believe they could get HIV no matter what their behavior including IDU and unprotected sex with men because they were not in a designated risk group. Sexual-orientation identity does not predict sexual behaviors.

Some women lacked basic knowledge about HIV such as how the virus gets from one body to another. Some believed that they must have tested negative for HIV because their Pap smears came out OK. Health care providers did not inform them of their sexual risks; no written educational materials were available for them, as were no products to decrease their risk. Many women were unsure of how and where to get reliable information about HIV and were ashamed that they did not already know. Very often, women had to educate sex partners about HIV and convince and cajole them about safer sex (Stevens, 1994).

A study of education of poor Haitian women in the Miami community found they had great difficulty in understanding several concepts central to HIV education in the biomedical tradition. Confusion about the meaning of positive (which meant good to these women) and negative (which meant bad to the women) persisted. Understanding of the antibody without symptoms, and of the window period between exposure and presentation of the antibody were also very difficult to comprehend. In their belief system, infection is signaled only by symptoms. Although Haitian populations in North American vary greatly in their proportions of acculturated and formally educated people, traditional beliefs will play a part in how people perceive AIDS and educational messages toward its prevention. Because many Haitian populations are at high risk of HIV infection, it is important to develop culturally effective educational programs for them (Wingerd & Page, 1997).

Survival for women following a diagnosis of AIDS is generally shorter than for men. Infected women typically present later for medical care than do men and present with more advanced disease, a higher rate of serious infection, more symptoms and a greater duration of symptoms. HIV-infected women have had less access to and less frequently accepted AZT, despite evidence of its effectiveness, including substantially reducing the risk of vertical transmission to the offspring of pregnant HIV-infected women.

A recent study revealed that negative attitudes toward use of AZT were widely prevalent in the African American and Puerto Rican communities. Women viewed the drug as highly toxic with distressing and dangerous side effects, prescribed indiscriminately, inadequately tested in women and inappropriate while women were feeling well. They believed that it typically did more harm than good to people who used it (Siegel & Gorey, 1997). Wider and more adherent use of AZT among women to both prolong survival and decrease the probability of vertical transmission will obviously require more patient education about treatment options. Because women place great faith in the experiential knowledge that others with the disease have acquired, peer counselors might be an excellent approach. These counselors would educate women about treatment options and encourage them to acknowledge potential benfits and weight them objectively against risks (Siegel & Gorey, 1997).

In general, a limited number of studies of educational programs about

HIV/AIDS directed toward the concerns of various groups of women as described previously, has been completed. In addition, some programs targeted to both women and men have been found to be less effective for participating women than for participating men, presumably because of limited emphasis on factors specific to HIV infection among women (Ickovics & Yoshikawa, 1998).

The majority of studies have a follow-up period of 6 months or less, and thus cannot address the sustained behavior necessary over long periods of time required for women in long-term relationships and those who wish to have children. Most use self-reported (and thus likely unreliable) condom use as the primary outcome. Both small-group and community-wide interventions have shown significant results (Ickovics & Yoshikawa, 1998). Peer-led interpersonal interventions focused on behavior change and incorporating gender-related influences have been found to be most effective (Wingood & DiClemente, 1996).

A review of 47 published studies of interventions for primary prevention of AIDS in women found programs that target women directly and include their gender and cultural issues, focus on behavioral skills and not just information, and include multiple sustained contacts can be effective in changing sexual risk behaviors. Interventions to maintain these behaviors are not yet well understood (Exner, Seal, & Ehrhardt, 1997).

An example of an innovative but as yet unevaluated intervention may be found in the program developed by Guthrie and others (1996) for prevention of HIV/AIDS and other sexually transmitted diseases in adolescent girls. The relationship between the theoretical constructs in Girl Talk and sample program activities may be found in Table 6.1. This peer-led intervention focuses on translation of knowledge into self-protective behavioral practices. It uses videotapes and interactive exercises to illustrate vulnerability, modeling, and the practice of self-protective behavior. Adolescent female development suggests that the illusion of invulnerability must be addressed and that effective learning is relational with peers. Full evaluation is ongoing.

Two studies of high-risk inner-city women provide examples of effective interventions. Each woman was individually assessed by a female assistant using a questionnaire and a sexual assertiveness skill role-playing task to ascertain risk behavior and other risk characteristics. The intervention included role-play of how each woman would respond to situations that required her to: initiate discussion of condom use, request that her partner postpone sex because he didn't have a condom, or refute her partner's protestations that condoms imply a lack of trust. To desensitize participants to issues involving condoms, condom demonstrations

TABLE 6.1 Theoretical Constructs As They Relate to Sample Activities in the Girl Talk Intervention

Theoretical construct	Sample program activities
Knowledge of benefits and barriers	A theme in the "Discover" and 'Express" sections, demonstrated by: 1. viewing breast self-exam videotape, discussions related to cost and consequences of not engaging in sex; 2. dialogue about things that would keep them from asking health professionals such as nurses to perform health-related activities such as pap tests or pelvic exams; 3. using female advanced nurse practitioners in adolescent health care; and 4. identifying behaviors over which participants have control, describing what risk means, reasons for continuing, and what they would need to help stop.
Perception of vulnerability	A theme in all three sections, demonstrated by: 1. sharing information related to sexually transmitted disease among adolescent females; 2. using peer groups as session facilitators: 3. explaining specific aspects of the female reproduction system that increase the likelihood of acquiring an infection (i.e.. a soft cervix and dark vaginal canal are good media for bacteria); and 4. using scenarios that explicate the relationship between vulnerable situations and increased risk (i.e., What If? scenarios).
Self-efficacy	A theme in the "Discover" and 'Express" sections, demonstrated by: 1. using the "Express Respect" video; 2. using peer-led facilitators helps participants see models similar to themselves solve problems successfully; 3. using What If? scenarios that reflect problems and situations in which participants may experience these problems; 4. using small groups of 8–10 participants; and 5. allowing time for role-playing specific refusal skills.
Sociocultural context	A theme in all three sections. demonstrated by: 1. using familiar names and places in scenarios; *(continued)*

TABLE 6.1 (Continued)

Theoretical construct	Sample program activities
	2. using peer-led groups: and 3. holding sessions at convenient places (e.g.. schools, recreational centers. housing projects) and times (before. during. or after school).

From Guthrie, B. J., Wallace, J., Doerr, K., Janz, N., Schottenfeld, D., & Selig, S. (1996). Girl talk: Development of an intervention for prevention of HIV/AIDS and other sexually transmitted diseases in adolescent females. *Public Health Nursing, 13,* 318–330. Reprinted by permission of Blackwell Science, Inc.

and practice with phallic replicas were incorporated in the sessions. Considerable attention was also directed toward identifying, understanding, and managing one's personal "triggers" to high-risk behavior, such as drinking or drug use, loneliness, or involvement in coercive or power-imbalanced sexual relationships. Group problem-solving approaches assisted participants in developing alternative strategies to handle situations that had formerly triggered high-risk sexual behavior. There were significant differences in the risk levels of sexual practices and condom-use patterns (Kelly et al., 1994).

With inner-city single pregnant women, Hobfoll, Jackson, Lavin, Britton, and Shepherd (1994) used video-taped segments featuring actors from a similar population illustrating assertiveness, negotiation, planning, and other skills such as cleaning drug works. Tapes served both as stimulus material and as models. Women imagined a scene in which they practiced an unhealthy behavior and had an aversive outcome such as becoming infected, to increase both a sense of vulnerability and mastery.

Educational programs aimed at learning to give self-care during HIV/AIDS illness or at women as caregivers of persons with AIDS could not be located in the literature. Measurement tools useful for assessment of patient need for education and for evaluation of educational programs are described in the text that follows.

EDUCATION FOR OTHER STDS IN WOMEN

Rates of curable STDs in the United States are the highest in the developed world and higher than in some developing regions. More than twelve million Americans, three million of whom are teenagers, are infected with STDs each year. The term "STD" denotes the more than 25 infectious organisms that are transmitted through sexual activity, along with the dozens of clinical syndromes they cause. The spectrum of health consequences ranges from mild acute illness to serious long-term complications such as cervical, liver, and other cancers and reproductive health problems (Eng & Butler, 1997).

Women and infants bear a disproportionate burden of STD-associated complications including infertility, ectopic pregnancy, chronic pelvic pain, and severe central nervous system damage and death in infants. Women are particularly vulnerable to STDs because they are more biologically susceptible and more likely to have asymptomatic infection that results in delayed diagnosis and treatment (Eng & Butler, 1997). Several studies of STD disease-related care seeking among adults and adolescents report that women delay care longer than do men. Difficulty in distinction of abnormal from normal genital discharges may explain this delay (Fortenberry, 1997).

An Institute of Medicine panel (Eng & Baker, 1997) called for a national initiative to increase knowledge and awareness of STDs, directed especially at adolescents before sexual activity is initiated. The lack of knowledge among women in high-risk groups is dramatic; 65% of young women reported almost no or very little knowledge about STDs (Eng & Baker, 1997). Knowledge is known to be important but not sufficient for change in behavior. Approaches for acquisition of safer sex behaviors were reviewed previously.

The developmental level of adolescent girls means that they may have difficulty with hypothetical thinking, making them vulnerable to poor judgment and unlikely to consider the long-term consequences of STD acquisiton. The personal fable, a belief that natural laws do not apply to oneself, occurs during the attainment of formal operational thinking. Adolescents often fail to recognize the signs and symptoms of STDs and may delay seeking health care even when they have had previous STD experience. Evidence suggests that adolescents do not understand asymptomatic infection (an abstract concept). This lack of comprehension is critical because STD transmission occurs through asymptomatic infection. For each adolescent, development is uneven across different domains, suggesting the importance of careful developmental assessment and using the adolescent's strengths in teaching and promoting adaptive choices (Baker & Rosenthal, 1998).

MEASUREMENT INSTRUMENTS

AIDS Knowledge, Feelings and Behavior Questionnaire

Developed by Barbara L. Dancy

The Aids Knowledge, Feelings and Behavior Questionnaire (AKFBQ) (Table 6.2) was developed as an ethnically sensitive and gender-specific questionnaire for African American women. It addresses sexual assertiveness. Little baseline data exist for this group even though they account for a significant percentage of female AIDS cases. This instrument is useful for effective planning and implementation of health promotion and prevention programs for this population. It can also be useful in stimulating discussion in self-help groups. Issues discussed might include difficulties women encounter in attempting to practice safer sex, and what support they can provide each other (Dancy, 1991).

Items were developed based on advice of the target population and health professions and piloted. The Knowledge subtest consists of 8 items measuring basic knowledge of AIDS and facts (question 1), and 16 items measuring knowledge of AIDS transmission and prevention (question 2). The Behavior subtest has 12 items that assess sexual behavior and substance-use behavior (questions 3 and 4) and six questions measuring sexual assertiveness (question 5). The Feeling subtest consists of seven items assessing AIDS stigmatization in the African American community (question 6). The internal consistencies (Cronbach's alphas) were: Knowledge subtest .66, Behavior subtest .84, and Feeling subtest .60 (Dancy, 1991).

Because all groups are heterogeneous in their understanding, it is important to know on what variables individuals differ. Further study with African American women showed that eductional level and age influenced their knowledge and attitudes about AIDS. For example, those with a college education knew that a person with the AIDS virus may appear completely well for months or years, that a positive HIV test is not synonymous with having AIDS, that a negative test doesn't imply immunity, that a person with the AIDS virus might not always develop the disease, that donating blood was not likely to result in transmission of AIDS, and other facts about transmission (Dancy, 1996).

Higher education had little influence on sexual behavior including assertive behavior. This finding is to be expected. Knowledge may not translate into risk-reduction behavior because people don't think the

TABLE 6.2   AIDS Knowledge, Feelings, and Behavior Questionnaire

Q-1 For the following, please indicate whether you agree or disagree with the statement. (Circle the number of your answer)

	Agree	Disagree	Don't Know
1. You can catch AIDS by being in the same room with a person who has AIDS or the AIDS-virus	1	2	8
2. AIDS is deadly disease	1	2	8
3. Symptoms of AIDS include loss of weight, diarrhea, tiredness, and pneumonia	1	2	8
4. A person with the AIDS-virus may appear to be completely well for months or years	1	2	8
5. If the AIDS test is negative (shows no sign of the AIDS-virus), the person is safe from getting AIDS	1	2	8
6. If a person's AIDS test is positive (shows signs of the AIDS-virus), it means the person has AIDS	1	2	8
7. A person with AIDS-virus will always develop AIDS	1	2	8
8. You can tell by looking at a person that he or she has AIDS	1	2	8

Q-2 For the following, please indicate whether the activity is very likely, somewhat likely, somewhat unlikely, or very unlikely to place a woman at risk of getting AIDS. (Circle the number of your answer)

	VERY LIKELY	SOMEWHAT LIKELY	SOMEWHAT UNLIKELY	VERY UNLIKELY	DON'T KNOW
1. Donate Blood	1	2	3	4	8
2. Share needles, syringes, and other "works" (drug equipment)	1	2	3	4	8
3. Have a blood transfusion	1	2	3	4	8
4. Use condoms (rubbers) or latex protection with every sex partner and every sexual act	1	2	3	4	8
5. Use sperm killing foam, cream or jelly containing nonoxynol-9 with every sex partner	1	2	3	4	8
6. Have sex with a man or a woman who used to shoot up drugs but doesn't shoot up anymore	1	2	3	4	8
7. Have sex with a man or a woman who has sex with a person who shoots up drugs	1	2	3	4	8

(continued)

TABLE 6.2 (Continued)

	VERY LIKELY	SOMEWHAT LIKELY	SOMEWHAT UNLIKELY	VERY UNLIKELY	DON'T KNOW
8. Have sex with a man who used to have sex with other men but no longer does	1	2	3	4	8
9. Have sex with a man with the AIDS virus	1	2	3	4	8
10. Have sex with a person who does not look sick but has the AIDS-virus	1	2	3	4	8
11. Have more than one sex partner within a six-month period	1	2	3	4	8
12. Have sex with no one	1	2	3	4	8
13. Have sex with only one man who doesn't have the AIDS-virus and who only has sex with you	1	2	3	4	8
14. Reduce the number of sex partners	1	2	3	4	8
15. Sit on toilet seats used by a person with AIDS or the AIDS-virus	1	2	3	4	8
16. Live or work with a person who has AIDS or the AIDS–virus	1	2	3	4	8

In order to develop effective AIDS educational programs specifically for African-american women, information is needed about the sexual and drug-use behavior of African-American women. Your answers will help us to develop these AIDS educational programs.

Q-3 Thinking back over the last 6 months, how often did you. . .

(Circle the number of your answer)

	ALL THE TIME	SOMETIMES	NEVER	NEVER, I'M MARRIED	NEVER, I'M NOT SEXUALLY ACTIVE
1. I have my own supply of condoms or latex protection	1	2	3	4	6
2. Leave it up to your partner to supply the condoms or latex protection	1	2	3	4	5

(continued)

TABLE 6.2   (Continued)

	ALL THE TIME	SOMETIMES	NEVER	NEVER, I'M MARRIED	NEVER, I'M NOT SEXUALLY ACTIVE
3. Let your partner decide if condoms or latex protection are to he used when you have sex	1	2	3	4	6
4. Avoid asking your partner to wear a condom or latex protection because your partner would get upset	1	2	3	4	6
5. Refuse to have sex with your partner if your partner didn't wear a condom or latex protection	1	2	3	4	6
6. Have your partner use a latex condom or latex protection with every sexual act	1	2	3	4	6

Q-4 In the last 6 months, I have. . .
(Circle the number of your answer)

	YES	NO
1. Had sex with only one man	1	2
2. Had sex with 2 or more men	1	2
3. Knowingly had sex with someone with AIDS or the AIDS-virus	1	2
4. Knowingly had sex with someone who had venereal disease	1	2
5. Used drugs or alcohol to get high	1	2
6. Shot up drugs	1	2

Q-5 Whether you are currently single, married, or in a long-term relationship, please consider the following situation: imagine that you meet a person with whom you would like to have sex, how likely is it that you would. . .
(Circle the number of your answer)

	MOST LIKELY	SOMEWHAT LIKELY	SOMEWHAT UNLIKELY	VERY UNLIKELY
1. Talk to person about your sexual likes and dislikes before you have sex	1	2	3	4

(continued)

TABLE 6.2 (Continued)

	MOST LIKELY	SOMEWHAT LIKELY	SOMEWHAT UNLIKELY	VERY UNLIKELY
2. Ask if a person has ever had sex with a man	1	2	3	4
3. Ask if a person has knowingly had sex with someone who uses drugs or alcohol to get high	1	2	3	4
4. Ask how often the person uses condoms or latex protection when having sex	1	2	3	4
5. Ask if the person has had any venereal diseases	1	2 ·	3	4
6. Ask if person shoots drugs	1	2	3	4

Q-6 For the following please indicate whether you strongly agree, agree, disagree or strongly disagree with the statement

(Circle the number of your answer)

	STRONGLY AGREE	AGREE	DISAGREE	STRONGLY DISAGREE	DON'T KNOW
1. AIDS is a curse	1	2	3	4	8
2. AIDS is a conspiracy (plan) against Black people	1	2	3	4	8
3. Anyone who gets AIDS deserves it, especially if the person is homosexual, bisexual, a prostitute, or a drug user	1	2	3	4	8
4. There should be no AIDS posters displayed in public	1	2	3	4	8
5. AIDS is a problem in the Black community	1	2	3	4	8
6. Homosexuality is a problem in the Black community	1	2	3	4	8
7. People with AIDS or the AIDS-virus should be allowed to prepare food for the public	1	2	3	4	8

From *American Journal of Health Behavior* (formerly *Health Values*) by Dancy, B. L., pp. 49–54. Copyright © 1991 PNG Publications. Reprinted with permission.

information applies to them or because people don't have the practical skills to supplement their abstract knowledge. Younger women were more likely to exhibit assertive sexual behaviors and to have fewer punitive attitudes toward people with AIDS. Education should be tailored to the group's understandings and behaviors, and demographic characteristics such as age and education are useful with this population (Dancy, 1996).

Contraceptive and Condom Decision Balance and Self-Efficacy Scales

Developed by Christine Galavotti

The Contraceptive and Condom Decision Balance and Self-Efficacy Scales (SE) (Table 6.3) measure two cognitive constructs central to the transtheoretical model of behavior change—decisional balance and self-efficacy. This theory posits that behavior change is a dynamic process of moving through five stages from precontemplation to action to maintenance of the behavior change. Decision-making theory suggests that people construct a balance sheet of comparative gains and losses. The balance is more heavily on the negative in the earlier stages of change and shifts to more predominantly positive in the action stage (Galavotti et al., 1995). Self-efficacy also should become stronger in later stages of behavior change.

The scales were piloted largely on a minority population. The means, standard deviations, and internal consistencies of each of the scales may be found on pages 125 and 126. For condom use with main partners, nearly half of the women were in the precontemplation stages, had no intention of changing in the forseeable future, and their decisional balance scores showed the cons outweighing the pros. For those in later stages, the pros dominated, providing evidence of validity for the test and generalizability of the transtheoretical model for this behavioral domain. This pattern has also been documented for a number of other behaviors such as smoking cessation.

These tools can provide the basis for a measure of program impact by documenting progress toward condom and contraceptive use and as a basis for developing intervention messages tailored to particular stages of behavior change. It offers a way to identify strategies that sway the decisional balance or enhance SE, or that are sensitive to a woman's readiness to change behavior.

TABLE 6.3   Decisional Balance and Self-Efficacy Scales

Characteristics of Decisional Balance Scales: Means, Standard Deviations, and Cronbach's Alphas

Scale item	M	SD
General contraceptive use		
Pros ($\alpha = .86$)		
1. I would be safer from pregnancy.	4.23	1.23
2. I would feel more responsible.	4.15	1.20
3. I would not have to deal with the results of a pregnancy,	4.27	1.23
4. I would be free to have sex without worrying about getting pregnant.	4.19	1.30
5. My partner would not have to worry about my becoming pregnant.	3.74	1.51
Cons ($\alpha = .81$)		
6. Birth control methods can make sex feel unnatural.	2.81	1.55
7. It would be too much trouble.	2.51	1.51
8. It would cost too much.	2.51	1.61
9. It is against my beliefs.	2.17	1.61
10. Sex would he less exciting	2.49	1.59
Condom use with main partner		
Pros ($\alpha = .93$)		
1. I would be safer from disease.	4.37	1.23
2. I would feel more responsible.	4.08	1.36
3. It protects my partner as well as myself.	4.35	1.27
4. I would be safer from pregnancy.	4.16	1.40
5. It is easily available.	4.22	1.27
Cons ($\alpha = .83$)		
6. It makes sex feel unnatural.	2.63	1.62
7. It would he too much trouble.	2.14	1.55
8. My partner would be angry.	2.36	1.60
9. I would have to rely on my partner's cooperation.	2.74	1.70
10. My partner would think that I do not trust him.	2.59	1.69
Condom use with other partners		
Pros ($\alpha = .82$)		
1. I would be safer from disease.	4.64	0.68
2. I would feel more responsible.	4.34	1.16
3. It protects my partner as well as myself.	4.54	0.98
4. I would be safer from pregnancy.	4.40	1.17
5. It is easily available.	4.22	1.27
Cons ($\alpha = .87$)		
6. It makes sex feel unnatural.	2.63	1.62
7. It would be too much trouble.	2.21	1.46
8. My partner would be upset.	2.22	1.52
9. My partner would think that I "play around."	2.34	1.62
10. I would have to rely on my partner's cooperation.	2.62	1.58

(continued)

TABLE 6.3   (Continued)

Characteristics of Self-Efficacy Scales: Means, Standard Deviations, and Cronbach's Alphas

Scale item	M	SD
General contraceptive use ($\alpha = .84$)		
"How confident are you that you would use. . ."		
1. When a method of birth control is not right on hand.	3.04	1.62
2. When you have been using alcohol or other drugs.	3.04	1.74
3. When your partner gets upset about it.	3.35	1.63
4. When you feel the side effects.	2.51	1.56
5. When it is too much trouble.	3.02	1.63
Condom use with main partner ($\alpha = .88$)		
"How confident are you that you would use. . ."		
1. When you have been using alcohol or other drugs.	2.88	1.71
2. When you are sexually aroused.	3.04	1.66
3. When you think your partner might get angry.	2.83	1.68
4. When you are already using another method of birth control.	2.94	1.66
5. When you want your partner to know you are committed to your relationship.	3.24	1.70
Condom use with other partners ($\alpha = .87$)		
"How confident are you that you would use. . ."		
1. When you think the risk for disease is low.	4.15	1.30
2. When you have been using alcohol or drugs.	3.72	1.51
3. When you are sexually aroused.	3.67	1.54
4. When you think your partner might get upset.	3.61	1.50
5. When you are already using another method of birth control.	3.68	1.52

Note. Scale scores for Decisional Balance Scales range from 1 = *not at all important* to 5 = *very important,* and for Self-Efficacy Scales, scale scores range from 1 = *not at all confident* to 5 = *extremely confident.*

From Galavotti, C., Cabral, R. J., Lansky, A., Grimley, D. M., Riley, G. E., & Prochaska, J. O. (1995). Validation of measures of condom and other contraceptive use among women at high risk for HIV infection and unintended pregnancy. *Health Psychology, 14,* 570–578.

A related tool—the Self-Efficacy Scale for HIV Risk Behaviors may be found in Smith, McGraw, Costa and McKinlay (1996). This tool focuses on risk behaviors of condom use, drug use with friends, and negotions with potential sexual partners. It was tested with a sample of young Latinos in two New England cities. Reliability coefficients (.77) were similar for men and women and both English-and Spanish-speaking respondents. Sexual experience, condom purchases and usage were positively related to SE as would be expected by the theory. In order to be effective, interventions must improve confidence in these abilities faster than this natural upward trend.

Empirical studies have consistently found perceived SE to be related to behavior change and maintenance. Many AIDS prevention programs have now embraced SE improvements as an intermediate goal in the effort to minimize the AIDS incidence.

SUMMARY

Educational programs for HIV/AIDS are poorly developed, consistent with the very slow medical response to the needs of women with these conditions. An immediately obvious characteristic of many of the approaches described in the literature is how male-oriented cultural assumptions about prevention make the educational task almost impossible (female responsibility for male condom use). Much of what is available about assessment of educational needs describes those of minority populations. More equitable solutions to problems faced by women in the HIV and STD epidemics are still needed.

REFERENCES

Baker, J. G., & Rosenthal, S. L. (1998). Psychological aspects of sexually transmitted infection acquisition in adolescent girls: A developmental perspective. *Developmental & Behavioral Pediatrics, 19,* 202–208.

Centers for Disease Control and Prevention. (1997). *HIV/AIDS Surveillance Report, 9(2),* 16, 37.

Cooper, E. B. (1995). Historical and analytical overview of policy issues affecting women living with AIDS: A bluprint for learning from our past. *Bulletin of the New York Academy of Medicine, 72*(Suppl. 1), 283–299.

Dancy, B. L. (1991). The development of an ethnically sensitive and gender-specific AIDS questionnaire for African-American women. *Health Values, 15*(6), 49–54.

Dancy, B. (1996). What African-American women know, do, and feel about AIDS: A function of age and education. *AIDS Education & Prevention, 8,* 26–36.

Eng, T. R., & Butler, W. M. (Eds). (1997). *The hidden epidemic.* Washington, DC: National Academy Press.

Exner, T. M., Seal, D. W., & Ehrhardt, A.A. (1997). A review of HIV interventions for at-risk women. *AIDS & Behavior, 1,* 93–124.

Fortenberry, J. D. (1998). Health care seeking behaviors related to sexually transmitted diseases among adolescents. *American Journal of Public Health, 87,* 417–420.

Galavotti, C., Cabral, R. J., Lansky, A, Grimley, D. M., Riley, G. E., & Prochaska, J. O. (1995). Validation of measures of condom & other contraceptive use among women at high risk for HIV infection and unintended pregnancy. *Health Psychology, 14,* 570–578.

Guthrie, B. J., Wallace, J., Doerr, K., Janz, N., Schottenfeld, D., & Selig, S. (1996). Gene talk: Development of an intervention for prevention of HIV/AIDS and other sexually transmitted diseases in adolescent females. *Public Health Nursing, 13,* 318–330.

Hobfoll, S. E., Jackson, A. P., Lavin, J., Britton, P. J., & Shepherd, J. B. (1994). Reducing inner-city women's AIDS risk activities: A study of single, pregnant women. *Health Psychology, 13,* 397–403.

Ickovics, J. R., & Hoshikawa, H. (1998). Preventive interventions to reduce heterosexual HIV risk for women: Current perspectives, future directions. *AIDS, 12*(Suppl. A), S197–S208.

Kelly, J. A., Murphy, D. A., Washington, C. D., Wilson, T. S., Koob, J. J., Davis, D. R., Ledezma, G., & Davantes, B. (1994). The effects of HIV/AIDS intervention groups for high-risk women in urban clinics, *American Journal of Public Health, 84,* 1918–1922.

O'Leary, A., Jemmott, L. S., Goodhart, F., & Gebelt, J. (1996). Effects of an institutional AIDS prevention intervention: Moderation by gender. *AIDS Education & Prevention, 8,* 516–528.

Siegel, K., & Gorey, E. (1997). HIV-infected women: Barriers to AZT use. *Social Science & Medicine, 45,* 15–22.

Smith, K. W., McGraw, S. A., Costa, L. A., & McKinlay, J. B. (1996). A self-efficacy scale for HIV risk behaviors: Development & evaluation. *AIDS Education & Prevention, 8,* 97–105.

Stevens, P. E. (1994). HIV prevention education for lesbians & bisexual women: A cultural analysis of a community intervention. *Social Science & Medicine, 39,* 1565–1578.

White, J. C. (1997). HIV risk assessment & prevention in lesbians & women who have sex with women: Practical information for clinicians. *Health Care for Women International, 18,* 127–138.

Wingerd, J. L., & Page, J. B. (1997). HIV testing among Haitian women: Lessons in the recognition of risk. *Health Education & Behavior, 24,* 736–745.

Wingood, G. M., & DiClemente, R. J. (1996). HIV sexual risk reduction interventions for women: A review. *American Journal of Preventive Medicine, 12,* 209–217.

Wortley, P. M., & Fleming, P. L. (1997). AIDS in women in the United States. *Journal of the American Medical Association, 278,* 911–916.

CHAPTER SEVEN

Other Disorders and Health Needs

T here are a number of other disorders that affect women significantly that seem to lack a tradition of education specifically focused on women's needs. These conditions include diabetes, arthritis, pain, and depression. Social expectations and roles, ways of learning and relating, physiology, and other variables guide special educational
opportunities for women. For some of these conditions there is little
research to elucidate the special needs of women, but this surely will
change.

DIABETES

Of adults with noninsulin-dependent diabetes mellitus (NIDDM), approximately 60% are women, with a disproportionate incidence in minority women (National Institutes of Health, 1995). The incidence of
diabetes in U. S. women is twice that of breast cancer. Among Black
women ages 65–74 the prevalence of NIDDM is 21%, which is the
highest incidence of diabetes of all Whites and Blacks (male and female) in all age categories. Prevalence of diabetes increases with ad-
vancing age in all racial and ethnic groups; approximately half of all
cases are in people older than 55 (Tinker, 1994). Insulin-dependent diabetes mellitus (IDDM) affects males and females equally.

In spite of the major investment in diabetes self-care management
education, there appears to be virtually no focus on the special experiences women may have with this disease beyond the reproductive area.
One might expect development of educational approaches particularly
focused for African American women, who are so heavily affected as a
group. Diabetic control fluctuates perceptibly in some girls and women

through the menstrual cycle, and menstrual function may be abnormal in times of poor diabetic control. Amenorrhea is the rule in untreated severe diabetes or following an attack of ketosis, when it may persist for several months (Nattrass, 1996). In addition, menstrual irregularity is quite common in women with diabetes. There is very little work on the interaction of menopause and diabetes, particularly on the effect of normal hormone fluctuations on blood glucose. Because women with diabetes are particularly at risk for coronary artery disease, the potential protective effect of hormone replacement therapy (HRT) would be of interest. Little information is available about HRT and diabetes. One medical center has made a commitment to include content related to menopause and special needs of women in their diabetes self-management program (Macdonald, 1997).

Of particular concern is the meticulous planning and management necessary from preconception until delivery for women with diabetes to deliver a healthy infant without detriment to their own health. The risks of spontaneous miscarriage as well as major congenital abnormality rise in proportion to the magnitude of elevation of the glycosylated hemoglobin. As organogenesis is complete by 7 weeks after conception, improvement in glycemic control after pregnancy has been confirmed is not sufficient to protect the fetus. Therefore, from puberty onward, all women with diabetes should be encouraged to plan each pregnancy, and it is essential that they are fully educated about why and how to manage contraception. Contrary to a widely held misconception, poor metabolic control does not impair fertility and should not be regarded as obviating the need for effective contraception (Kenshole, 1997).

Intentional insulin omission, frequently used as a means of weight management but occurring sometimes because the individual was overwhelmed by diabetes, was reported by about one third of women with IDDM, as studied by Polonsky and others (1994). Omission generally occurred on an infrequent basis with only 9% of the total subject sample reporting frequent omission. Omitters evidenced poorer glycemic control, more diabetes-related hospitalizations, and higher rates of retinopathy and neuropathy. Although rates of omission seemed to peak during late adolescence and early adulthood, they remained markedly elevated through adulthood. The health-care team should prepare the patient for the temporary weight gain that often accompanies improving glycemic control. Those who consistently omit insulin for weight management might well be referred to a mental-health practitioner who is knowledgeable about diabetes and disordered eating (Polonsky et al., 1994)

Study of IDDM among children ages 0–18 and excluding pregnancy-related diagnoses, showed that females had 40% more hospitalizations and 44% more repeat hospitalizations than did males. Although hospitalizations do not capture the full spectrum of diabetes-related morbidity, hospital use is one proxy measure for morbidity resulting from IDDM. Both acute and chronic diabetes complications that require hospitalization are associated with poor glucose control. Gender differences occurred primarily in adolescents and were observed for diabetic ketoacidosis. These findings suggest that glucose control may not have been as good in females. This may occur because of poorer compliance, biological factors that make glucose control more difficult in young women such as changes in glucose metabolism during the menstrual cycle, or because of insulin omission and disordered eating (Cohn, Cirillo, Wingard, Austin, & Roffers, 1997).

Many of the qualitative studies pertaining to the experiencing of diabetes have been conducted with well-educated, female Caucasians who have IDDM and who live with an friend or helper (Paterson, Thorne, & Dewis, 1998). Living with diabetes required compromises between breaks from and compliance with the medical regimen. At a turning point in living with diabetes, many patients made a conscious decision to assume control, frequently precipitated by recognizing that compliance with prescribed regimens did not prevent diabetes-related complications. Learning to know their bodily cues and basic knowledge about diabetes formed the base for developing an appropriate regime of diet, exercise, and medication. Patients also accepted that perfection is impossible because bodily responses are not always predictable.

Individuals who successfully manage their diabetes take "breaks" from active self-care occasionally, by testing less or not at all and eating foods not on the prescribed diet. These breaks are viewed as helping to maintain a sense of self-control. Health care professionals must not assume that the decision to control is permanent and recognize that it can change with variations in life events and the disease itself. The studies suggested that recruitment of "allies" is critical to diabetes self-care management. These persons must be educated for diabetes care in order to play their important roles and to understand the individual's unique responses and strategies (Paterson et al., 1998).

Although there are many measurement tools available for diabetes self-management (Bradley, 1994; Redman, 1998), their measurement characteristics and norms with populations of women apparently have been infrequently studied.

One study has shown gender differences in the Diabetes Attitude Scale (Fitzgerald, Anderson, & Davis, 1995). Women were more likely to view NIDDM as a serious disease and to believe that it has a negative impact on the patient's life (Fitzgerald et al., 1995). Because patients who reported high adherence levels had more favorable attitudes toward diabetes, it may be worth checking this relationship with women as well as understanding why women experienced diabetes more negatively. Few differences were observed in the recommendations reported by patients to have been given by health professionals to men and women, and in adherence to the components of self-care.

In summary, self-management education for women with diabetes needs to vary according to their developmental status and should differ in some ways from that of men. In the adolescent, peer acceptance is closely related to the girl's self-acceptance of her body image and self-esteem. The higher incidence of eating disorders among young women and the fact that for those with diabetes these disorders can be life-threatening and are correlated significantly with poorer levels of glycemic control, is one special area. During early and middle adulthood, marital relationships, family life and the decision whether to have children may all be affected by diabetes. The dearth of literature regarding management of sexual problems in women with diabetes is problematic and should be an area of educational focus. This is consistent with the general tendency to ignore the sexual implications of physical illness in women. Issues regarding contraception and pregnancy are more commonly acknowledged (Hartman-Stein & Reuter, 1988).

ARTHRITIS

The autoimmune diseases are more common in women than men. Virtually any organ system of the female anatomy can be affected by these illnesses. Actual prevalence ranges from the high of 10–15 females for each male with systemic lupus erythematosis to four females for every male with rheumatoid arthritis (RA). In women, the most common chronic health condition is arthritis. RA affects women three times more often than men, although the incidence in younger women compared with younger men is closer to 5:1. The course of the disease is unpredictable and can range from very mild with limited involvement of joints to severe deformities affecting multiple joints (Dwyer, 1997). Most investigators suspect that the signs and symptoms of the diseases vary with the menstrual cycle and improve during pregnancy with exacerbation postpartum (Case & Reid, 1998; Lahita, 1996).

Most forms of arthritis are not preventable. Changes in health behaviors are generally unrelated to the occurrence, remission, and exacerbation of rheumatic disease (Goeppinger & Lorig, 1996). Learning to cope with pain, the most common symptom of RA appears to be key in promoting health status, with self-efficacy enhancing interventions especially important (Dwyer, 1997). Shaul's (1995) studies of women learning to live with RA describe how self-efficacy develops. The women described four distinct stages, beginning with awareness and proceeding to mastery, although some had not achieved the final stage. After awareness in which the hope was that symptoms would be transitory and that their strength and agility would be restored, "getting care" was characterized by being overwhelmed by symptoms of pain, stiffness, joint swelling, fatigue, and depression. "Shopping" for a doctor and trial-and-error treatment were common experiences.

After diagnosis, the women were told by physicians that they "would just have to learn to live with it." This period was characterized by a sense of isolation, of being out of touch with others, and of having symptoms taken lightly by physicians, family members, and friends. The next flare usually could not be predicted, and the disease and its symptoms assumed a dominant place in their daily lives as the women attempted to attend to self-care needs, role responsibilities, and relationships. They learned to listen to their bodies to recognize cues of oncoming flares, learned how to titrate medications to obtain the best effect, when to exercise and when to stop, as well as when to rest and when to keep moving. They tried to keep a positive attitude and asked others for help.

At the mastery stage, they were able to incorporate the disease and its symptoms into everyday life and recognize the cues that signalled the onset of a flare, overwork, or the need to change a pattern of activity. Through the acquisition of knowledge about the disease, its treatment and the experience of living with it, they developed a level of expert insight. Mastery involved learning how to reset goals and expectations, how to ask for and receive help from others, how to marshal and manage one's energy, how to maintain connections with family and community without becoming depleted, and how to work with the physician in managing medical routines. Mastery is similar to normalization; the individual redefines what constitutes normal and no longer sees the illness as something temporary (Shaul, 1997).

Health care workers were seldom cited as providing the support the women felt was needed in the early years of living with RA (Shaul, 1995). Why? .

Although there have been 20 years of arthritis patient-education research, with the Arthritis Self-Management Program (ASMP) well established in the United States and used throughout the world, a summary of this work as it relates to women could not be located. A general summary of this research shows that study samples were predominantly comprised of Caucasian and middle-aged-to-elderly women with osteoarthritis and individuals with 12 or more years of schooling. Short-and long-term improvements in pain and depression as well as in self-efficacy and helplessness have been demonstrated. Subsequent studies are testing these interventions with ethnic minority groups (Goeppinger & Lorig, 1996).

The ASMP is a community-based program using peer educators that is heavily focused on development of self-efficacy. It aims to enhance perceived ability to control various aspects of arthritis through skills mastery, modeling, reinterpretation of symptoms, and persuasion. Participants are also active learners in problem-solving groups who self-contract for behavioral changes. Decreases in feelings of helplessness and increases in self-efficacy rather than changes in self-care behaviors are associated with improvements (Goeppinger & Lorig, 1996).

A study of the ASMP with a sample of 94% women with a mean disease duration of RA or osteoarthritis (OA) of 26 years found that after 4 months, participants demonstrated not only significant increases in self-efficacy but also in positive affect, cognitive symptom management, communication with physicians, exercise, and relaxation. The study design did not include a comparison group (Barlow, Williams, & Wright, 1997).

A clinical trial of a concise program of self-care education delivered as an adjunct to primary care for inner-city patients with knee osteoarthritis (Mazzuca et al., 1997) found notable preservation of function and control of resting knee pain. The group studied was 85% women and 69% African American, with an average of 9.7 years of formal education. The education was delivered by an arthritis nurse specialist in one instructional session with follow-up phone calls that is considerably more abbreviated than the ASMP. The instruction emphasized the nonpharmacologic management of joint pain, preservation of function by problem solving, and the practice of behavioral principles of joint protection. A summary of knowledge questionnaires, attitude measures, and an arthritis self-efficacy scale may be found in Redman (1998).

PAIN

Women are more likely than men to experience a variety of recurrent pains. In most studies women report more severe levels of pain, more frequent pain, and pain of longer duration than do men. Women have moderate or severe pain from menstruation (75% of late adolescent females), pregnancy, and childbirth including chronic episiotomy pain. Although neither men nor women appear to receive adequate analgesia, there is suggestive evidence that women receive even less adequate analgesia from providers. The findings from research studies on gender differences in responses to painful stimuli and analgesic medications suggest that men and women do respond differently to both pain and pain medications (Unruh, 1996). Females suffer more than do males from migraine and cluster headaches, trigeminal neuralgia, carpal tunnel syndrome, and temporomandibular joint disorder (Miaskowski, 1997).

Females suffer from a larger number of chronic pain syndromes and live longer with chronic pain and disability. Decreased socialization, falls, slow rehabilitation, cognitive dysfunction, malnutrition, depression, sleep disturbance, impaired ambulation, and polypharmacy have all been associated with the presence of pain among elderly persons (Turk, Okifuji, & Scharff, 1994).

These syndromes are particularly problematic for elderly women. Twenty-five to 50% of community-dwelling older adults suffer as a result of chronic pain problems, and among nursing home residents, where women predominate, prevalence of pain is even higher (45%–80%). Cancer, osteoarthritis, and osteoporosis, which commonly afflict women, cause pain. Within the limited geriatric pain literature, virtually no direct attention is given to chronic pain among older women even though it limits activities of daily living, is a major source of anxiety, and contributes to feelings of stress and burden (Roberto, 1994).

The prevalence of chronic pelvic pain of at least 6 months' duration, its cause frequently undiagnosed, was found in a population-based study to have a prevalence of 14.7% in women aged 18 to 50 (Mathias, Kupperman, Liberman, Lipschutz, & Steege, 1996). This literature shows that women's pain burden is significant and that its impact on the quality of their lives is significant.

Determining the mechanisms underlying these gender differences may provide insight into use of different assessment tools and pain-management strategies for men and women (Miaskowski, 1997). While pain assessment is considered to be an essential aspect of treatment, little research has delineated factors relevant to such assessment for geriatric women suffering from chronic pain (Turk et al., 1994). Therefore, appropriate normative information may be unavailable, making conclusions about the pain these patients are experiencing difficult to draw.

Educating the patient and family that pain is not a normal part of aging (Roberto, 1997) seems duplicitous unless help in relieving that pain is available. In general, education for chronic pain is a very under-developed area; the degree to which it is made available and what its content is is largely undescribed.

Ferrell and others do describe pain-management education for elderly patients with cancer at home (Ferrell, Ferrell, Ahn, & Tran, 1994). The teaching was conducted during three home visits over a 2-week time period. Included was general information about pain, use of pain rating scales, pharmacologic and nonpharmacologic intervention with demonstration of these techniques. Audiotape reinforcement was provided. Improvement in knowledge and experience were reported. Description and critique of the Patient Pain Questionnaire, its development and use may be found in Redman (1998) as well as in original sources. Structured pain education should be provided to all patients with cancer who experience this symptom (Ferrell et al., 1994).

Evaluation of interventions to treat chronic pain focuses not only on the amount of pain relieved but also on the extent to which functional status is enhanced. Yet, measures of activity level are based on the assumption that a given list of activities is equally important to both genders and frequently does not include child care or other care-taking activities, and few studies have looked at gender differences in functional status. Vallerand (1998) describes development and psychometric evaluation of the Inventory of Functional Status—Chronic Pain (IFS-CP), an instrument developed to measure functional status in women with chronic pain. The tool includes performance of the usual household, social and community activities, child care, care of parents or dependent family members, personal care, as well as occupational and educational activities. Functional status instruments developed for the general population may include questions that are not relevant for women, but more important, may not assess activities engaged in primarily by women. This is particularly the case for child and home care, roles many women retain even if they work outside the home. Such inclusions are likely to provide a more comprehensive understanding of the effects of chronic pain on the lives of women.

Items for the IFS-CP were generated from reports from women with chronic pain, and women with chronic pain seeking treatment at an anesthesia pain center served as content validity judges. This choice of judges is admirable and reflects the belief that patients, not providers, are best able to identify activities most relevant in their lives. The instrument has good initial psychometric characteristics but must be tested with a broader range of populations of women beyond highly educated Caucasian women between 20 and 60 years of age (Vallerand, 1998).

Pain, acute but especially chronic, is an area of profound impact on women's lives with a significant effect on functional status and quality of life. Development of appropriate measurement tools and educational programs is of great importance.

DEPRESSION AND ANGER

Depression—an unpleasant feeling of sadness and dejection marked by difficulty in sleeping, concentrating, and acting—is at least twice as common in women as in men. A female preponderance is evident from puberty on and found across a range of time, cultures, and countries. In the month after childbirth, there is a 22-fold increase in the incidence of affective psychoses with the main trigger thought to be neurophysiological. There is also a less dramatic rise in nonpsychotic depression thought to relate more to psychosocial stressors. It is believed that social factors such as childhood sexual abuse, low self-esteem (Meagher & Murray, 1997), and unequal adult social status with men play a role in these differences. Women's levels of depression diminish as their work and family circumstances approach those more typical for males, whose patterns have formed the norm (Mirowsky, 1996).

Education can serve several important functions for women with depression. Frederickson and Roberts (1997) describe educational efforts flowing from objectification theory, which posits that girls and women are typically acculturated to internalize an observer's perspective as a primary view of their physical selves. Sexual objectification is but one form of gender oppression. It is the experience of being treated as a body, valued predominantly for its use to others. This perspective on self can lead to habitual body monitoring, which can increase women's opportunity for shame and anxiety, reduce opportunities for peak motivational states, and diminish awareness of internal bodily states.

The theory hypothesizes that accumulation of such experiences helps account for an array of mental health risks such as unipolar depression, sexual dysfunction, and eating disorders, which disproportionately affect women. The experiences combine to create an experience women describe as "loss of self"—trying to be the way another person wants you to be instead of the way you are. Education makes women aware of these dynamics and the adverse psychological effects they can have and teaches them to resist these cultural messages and experience their bodies in positive ways (Frederickson & Roberts, 1997). Education can also be aimed at reducing abuse and violence toward women, encouraging childraising practices that promote equal treatment for boys and girls, and supporting equal opportunity in education and occupation (Sprock & Yoder, 1997).

Burnside and Hodgins (1992) describe the use of education in a social network intervention designed to treat clinically depressed older women called the Social Health Outreach Program (SHOP). SHOP takes the position that depression among women should frequently be interpreted as a state of demoralization caused by a social identity deficit resulting from a role-determined construction of opportunities. Social isolation is believed to be structured into the traditional female role.

Participants learn that the way to deal with the problem is to develop competency for self-management. The educational component provides participants with information that enables them to construct a rationale for changing their social worlds in specific ways. This approach empha-sizes a collaborative, participatory teaching–learning process that en-gages learners in the creation of knowledge based on personal experience that can be used as the basis for individual change and social action. In SHOP, education functions as a tool for perspective transformation, dur-ing which participants are sensitized to "blame-the-victim" biases inher-ent in psychological and medical approaches to treating depression (Burnside & Hodgins, 1992).

So SHOP was developed to challenge psychiatry's view that women who are not happy in their traditional roles must be sick. It holds that women's high risk of depression is a social, not medical problem. Like a similar intervention by Gordon and Ledray (1986), SHOP includes information sharing, skills training for positive thinking and assertive-ness, experiential learning, and intellectual stimulation. Participants learn how to construct a satisfactory social self through community participa-tion. Both interventions show a significant reduction in depression among participants, although Burnside and Hodgins do not regard SHOP's ed-ucational dimension as primary therapy for depression.

Congruent with the notion of capabilities to perform mental-health-related self-care, West and Isenberg (1997) have developed a tool based on Orem's theory, to measure such capabilities. The Mental Health relat-ed Self-Care Agency Scale (MH-SCA) measures the ability to maintain attention and exercise vigilance with respect to self as self-care agent; controlled use of available energy; motivation; ability to make decisions about care of self, and ability to acquire technical knowledge about self-care; repertoire of cognitive, perceptual, manipulative, communication, and interpersonal skills; ability to order discrete self-care actions; and ability to consistently perform self-care operations. Content validity has been supported, the scale discriminated between depressed and nondepressed women, and internal consistency was .90 (West & Isenberg, 1997).

Questions have been raised about both diagnostic criteria for depression and scales for measurement of depression. Do they adequately reflect men's experience of depression (Sprock & Yoder, 1997), and do they contribute to "overdiagnosis" of depression among women?

A small but interesting body of literature has been developed to address anger and its expression in women. Women's anger arises in their closest relationships and is a response to conditions of disrespect and injustice, irresponsibility of others, and powerlessness to get someone or something to change. The inability to make oneself heard, perhaps the epitome of powerlessness, is an especially hurtful anger precipitant. In American society, anger is freely expressed by individuals in positions of power and dominance but denied expression in subordinates, with differences by culture and region of the country (Thomas, 1998). A small qualitative study of African American women in the southern United States found that they were more often empowered by their anger than defeated by it, perhaps because of different socialization than that experienced by Caucasian women (Fields et al., 1998).

Anger can become problematic when it is too frequent, too intense, too prolonged, or managed ineffectively. Women are more likely than are men to suppress their anger, taking no overt action perhaps because expressing it does not conform to the feminine ideal of the selfless, ever-nurturing person and creates fear of rejection or disruption in relationships that women consider vital to their well-being (Thomas, 1995). There is a growing body of evidence that this pattern is related to elevated blood pressure, which is a significant health problem for women, especially as they age (Thomas, 1997). Other health problems thought to be associated with unhealthy ways of handling anger include depression, eating disorders, and smoking (Droppelman, Thomas, & Wilt, 1995).

Teaching about healthy anger is one of the intervention strategies that can be used. Many people gain insight by keeping an anger log or diary and analyzing it for patterns. Patients can be taught to take contructive action on the precipitants of anger, making an assertive request and bargaining to resolve a problem. Anger-prone women may need to modify unrealistic expectations regarding their own behavior or that of other people. In situations in which no constructive action is possible, people can be taught to use distraction techniques or physically discharge anger arousal through vigorous physical exercise. Behavioral practice with role playing should be part of the intervention plan (Thomas, 1998). Such interventions are perhaps most important for those women with chronic stressors and/or high levels of trait anger and irrational cognitions (Thomas, 1995). Thomas (1995) believes that many measurement instruments include behaviors more characteristic of men and not including approaches such as rational discussion of anger, shown in several studies to be preferred by women.

GENDER AS A RISK FACTOR FOR ADVERSE EVENTS WITH MEDICATIONS

Women are far more likely than are men to experience adverse reactions to prescribed drugs and twice as likely to die from side effects as men, possibly because the dosage levels have been determined by testing in men. Dose and duration of action of a drug may depend significantly on the sex of the patient. For example, although most studies delineating the optimal dosages of psychotropically active substances have been done on men, 70% of prescriptions for such medications are written for women. Even after weight and age matching of subjects, women have higher plasma levels of psychotropic drugs, especially if they are on oral contraceptives (Legato, 1997).

Gender-specific pharmacokinetics studies (which study absorption, distribution, metabolism, and elimination of drugs) are largely absent in the literature. Numerous examples of limited data indicating areas of concern from not understanding how common drugs act during various phases of the menstrual cycle, pregnancy, lactation, contraception, and during menopause with and without HRT, may be found in Berg (1997). Looking at some of what is known shows the significant potential for errors in drug management in women. Drug absorption can be altered at different stages of the menstrual cycle. Oral contraceptives can significantly influence and be influenced by metabolism of others drugs, yielding contraceptive failure. Dose regimens appropriate for nonpregnant patients are still widely used in pregnant women even though pregnancy commonly brings reduction in the gastric emptying rate. Increase in hepatic clearance and renal elimination of certain drugs during pregnancy is acknowledged (Xie, Piecoro, & Wermeling, 1997).

Differences between the sexes in drug absorption occurs in several routes of administration. Women empty solids from the stomach more slowly than do men, which affects the availability of a drug for systemic absorption. Gastric pH is higher in women than men, which decreases the gastric absorption of weak acid drugs. Because women have a higher proportion of adipose tissue than men, drugs delivered intramuscularly may be deposited in fat and absorbed more slowly from it. Drug absorption in the lungs also may be influenced by sex. Drugs of the same pharmacologic class may show markedly different effects by sex. The liver is the primary organ responsible for drug metabolism and chemical detoxification. Sex differences have been observed with many drugs that undergo hepatic metabolism.

Some antidepressant drugs may create adverse effects in infants of breast-feeding mothers. Women have been found to experience more bleeding episodes after thrombolytic therapy. Women also respond to antihypertensive treatment differently (Xie et al., 1997).

In summary, there are a number of examples of sex differences in drug pharmacokinetics and pharmacodynamics. Although the clinical significance of many sex differences in drug metabolism remains to be determined (Harris, Benet, & Schwartz, 1995), findings that are reliable should not only be incorporated into practice but into drug information and patient-education programs.

EPILEPSY

In epilepsy, seizures are often linked to menarche, the menstrual cycle, and menopause. Up to 70% of women with epilepsy claim that most of their seizures are exacerbated by menstruation, perhaps related to cyclic alterations in both ovarian hormone levels and drug metabolism. The sex hormones alter the excitability of neurons in the cerebral cortex, with estrogens lowering the seizure threshold and progestins having the opposite effect and protecting against seizures (Case & Reid, 1998; Liporace, 1997).

There is a high failure rate of hormonal contraception in women taking hepatic enzyme-inducing antiepileptic drugs. During pregnancy, seizures can negatively affect fetal development and antiepileptic drugs are associated with an increased risk of congenital anomalies in the offspring. Thus, good seizure control is important. So too is monitoring of antiepileptic drug levels during pregnancy and postpartum because drug levels decline as a result of changes in liver metabolism, renal clearance, volume of distribution and abosrption, and return to baseline by 12 weeks after delivery. At menopause, more than half of women experience a change in seizure frequency (Liporace, 1997). It is essential that epilepsy education programs include content and skills specific to the needs of women.

ASTHMA

Several interesting sex/gender differences in diagnosis and management of asthma have been reported but at this time it is not clear what their relevance for patient education is for girls and women.

In children, asthma has been believed to be more prevalent in boys than in girls, with the sex ratio changing in the adult years. Several biological explanations for these differences have been developed. A cultural explanation has also been suggested based on the observation that prevalence of asthma-like symptoms was similar in 13- and 14-year-old boys and girls in France. Underdiagnosis in girls and under-treatment of diagnosed female cases of childhood asthma may be a partial answer to the sex ratio in prevalence (Berlier, Burel, Lanteaume, Veruloet, & Charpin, 1997).

Most studies report a female preponderance in the use of health care in treatment of asthma (medication, clinical services, and admission to hospital). It is not clear if this is caused by differences in prevalence, severity, or management of the disease. In a study in which hospital admissions for asthma were adjusted for the underlying prevalence of self-reported asthma and smoking, women had an approximately 70% higher risk of being admitted to hospital than did men. Clinical studies have indicated that women may have inadequate inhaler technique and physicians may be reluctant to prescribe steroids for women because of the possibility of pregnancy or concern for potential bone demineralization (Prescott, Lange, Vestbo & The Copenhagen City Heart Study Group, 1997).

Menstrual-linked asthma (MLA) was been detected in about a fourth of female asthmatics in one study and appears to represent a more severe form of the disease. It was associated with an increase in airway resistance and not simply the result of an increased perception of symptoms during the premenstrual or menstrual weeks. It has been described as a cause of repeated hospitalizations, recurrent respiratory failure, and even death. The exact pathophysiology of MLA is unknown. History taking should include questions related to menstrual variation of asthma. These patients need to be monitored more closely and educated about initiation of appropriate preventive measures to better control their asthma (Agarwal & Shah, 1997). Another study has shown that long-term and/or high doses of postmenopausal hormone therapy increase subsequent risk of adult-onset asthma in women (Troisi et al., 1995).

A study by Osborne, Vollmer, Linton, & Buist (1998) found that women with asthma reported more symptoms and experienced poorer quality of life than did men even though objective measures of airflow did not differ. These women reported use of more health care and more medications for asthma than did men. The data suggest that men and women respond differently to their asthma. Although there are no data confirming that focusing asthma education on women would decrease health care usage, the authors believe it seems a reasonable first step.

In summary, potential underdiagnosis, higher hospitalization rates, symptoms and quality of life, and menstrual-related exacerbations of asthma characterize asthma care for women.

EATING DISORDERS

Lifetime prevalence of bulimia nervosa (BN) in women is 4%–8%, with increasing prevalence among young women (Treasure et al., 1994). Although psychological treatment is thought to be the most successful of the options available, group psychoeducation has also been studied with excellent results in decreasing binge eating and vomiting among those who are not severely symptomatic. Frequently the instruction is delivered in part by use of self-help manuals structured according to behavioral skills training including self-monitoring, goal setting, assertiveness, cognitive restructuring, problem solving, and strategies to prevent relapse. Treatment is directed at the interruption of target symptoms, the normalization of eating, examination of the 'function' of symptoms, learning to cope with situations that lead to symptomatic behavior, and the identification of thoughts, beliefs, and values that perpetuate eating problems (Olmsted et al., 1991).

In addition, patients with eating disorders have considerable misconceptions about dieting, weight regulation, nutrition, and the physical and mental consequences of their disorder, which can also be addressed by education. Many behavioral treatment packages incorporate these educational components (Schmidt, Ali, Sloane, Tiller, & Treasure, 1995).

Although several studies do not indicate the sex composition of their study samples, the study designs are not randomized controlled trials, and temporary fluctuations in symptom severity are common in these patients (Cooper, Coker & Fleming, 1994; 1996; Thiels, Schmidt, Treasure, Garthe, & Troop, 1998), these studies using supervised psychoeducation and manuals have now shown significant therapeutic results. If these findings hold up, they offer the opportunity to provide help more cheaply to more patients including those in primary care settings (Olmsted et al., 1991).

Friedman (1998) has developed an eating disorder prevention program for preadolescent/adolescent girls. The program validates girls' experiences and feelings, reframes them in terms of female development and provides girls with an understanding of the societal pressures they face. The program has not yet been evaluated.

CAREGIVING

Traditionally and still today women play the role of principal health care brokers of the American family. Women are more likely than are men to seek and use health care, possess greater knowledge about health, be compliant with a therapeutic regimen, and monitor the health and safety of others as well as their own health (Norcross, Ramirez, & Palinkas, 1996). Two thirds to three quarters or more of all family caregivers are women (Candib, 1995). Nearly half of the caregivers surveyed have been in this role for 6 years or more (Stensland, 1998).

It is generally assumed that any woman can give care with little or no formal training, and to the extent taught, this care is modeled on that given by one's mother. Indeed, health policy is based on the implicit assumption that women are available to provide care in the home, and recent policy requires even more of this investment by families and women.

Feminists believe that this system is oppressive to many women and that health professionals are complicit in sustaining it. Males dominate the political and economic institutions that make this policy, and care is dependent on the caregiving work done by women, with limited social recognition (Covan, 1997). The system of control can extend to sanctions against a caregiver if she cannot demonstrate competence to health professionals' standards. In such a circumstance, a mother can be judged unfit and a child removed from her care.

Much of the literature focuses on emotional outcomes and burdens of care provision, an imbalance of demands relative to resources available. There is less focus on the positive aspects of seeing caregiving as making one's link in the chain of reciprocity. It is clear that social support buffers the stress of caregiving and that caregivers with lower income report more distress, depression, and less satisfaction (Candib, 1995). Many caregivers are faced with gaining very complex skills in management of sophisticated technologies for health conditions and transferring them into the home setting. These include dialysis, nutrition, ventilation, and infusion technologies. Lack of coordination of services, training, information, financial assistance, and ability to plan for the future have been cited as problematic for these families. Studies show that long-term emotional adjustments of caregivers and their patients are related to problem solving ability; yet, no studies were found in which techniques of problem-solving were taught. Neither were longitudinal studies available, describing caregiver learning needs over time. Follow-up and re-training needs during caregiving are also important (Smith, 1996).

There is little evidence that families know how to implement care effectively. The outcomes of family caregiving are very rarely addressed. To what extent does home care facilitate or hinder recovery of function or successful adaptation to impairments experienced by the elderly? Do caregivers do what care recipients really need? Can they effectively provide therapeutic and rehabilitative as well as custodial care? Do confidence and preparedness alter caregivers' reactions? How are caregiving skills including decision-making skills acquired? How do processes of care change across time as caregivers master the tasks and adapt to the role? Do education and training demonstrate significant impact on caregivers' behavior or beliefs or responses to giving care? Which caregivers are more likely to respond to which interventions (Given, 1991)?

Most research has been focused on the negative impact that caregiving has imposed, with much focus on caregiver burden. A pervasive sense of not knowing what to expect or how to interpret what is happening as well as the open-ended nature of the caring process leads to strain among caregivers. Positive feelings, including increased self-esteem from feelings of competence and fulfillment of social roles, have emerged as significant predictors of less stressful caregiving experiences (Given & Given, 1991).

Generic caregiver support programs provide three components. Educational activities focus on nurture and self-care, enhancement of self-esteem, stresses of caregiving, and effects of chronic illness on family functioning. Caregivers are taught stress-reduction methods, assertiveness training, problem solving, health-promotion techniques, and legal and financial issues. Emotional health activities include group counseling, support experiences, and coping skills to deal with grief and loss, loneliness, role reversal, denial, and anger. Directed activities include relaxation techniques and stimulation of leisure-time activities such as arts and crafts (Kleffel, 1998).

Research has shown that psychoeducational interventions with caregivers can be effective. A review of six studies of such interventions for caregivers of persons with dementia found outcomes of increased social support, decreased depression, decreased burden and improved knowledge about dementia care (Collins, Givens, & Givens, 1994).

Caregiver organizations that are sources of services, printed information, and Internet resources are described by Stensland (1998).

Three specific examples of caregiver education are considered here. First, Ferrell, Grant, Chan, Ahn, and Ferrell (1995) provide the same education described previously for caregivers of elderly cancer patients in pain, 76% of whom were female. The Family Pain Questionnaire, which parallels the Patient Pain Questionnaire, is also described and critiqued in Redman (1998) as well as in original sources. It measures knowledge of pain principles and of medication, experiences with the patient's pain, and caregiver roles in pain relief. The tool has been shown to be sensitive to educational intervention.

Second, Conley and Burman (1997) describe needs of family caregivers living in rural areas and their frustrating attempts to obtain information. They needed information about the underlying reason for symptoms; the patient's disease progression; treatment options and side effects; what symptoms to expect now and in the future; and learning needs in ambulation, bowel management, comfort care, dietary control, pain management or wound and skin care and supportive services. Two thirds of these caregivers were female. Although they were aggressive in seeking information, pamphlets were of little help and physicians were not accessible for information or help. Although these caregivers turned to informal sources, the lack of access to educational services led to frustration, anxiety, and inability to make decisions about care. Home care nurses can play a critical role in helping caregivers develop formal and informal networks of support.

Wife and daughter caregivers for patients with Alzheimer's disease were taught specific skills to manage anger and frustration more effectively in their caregiving situations (Gallagher-Thompson & DeVries, 1994). Details may be found in their article. These skills included learning to relax in very stressful situations, techniques for identifying and challenging dysfunctional thoughts that trigger angry feelings, and assertiveness communication skills with the frail elder and other family members. These were skills women caregivers frequently did not have. Each week, participants practiced the new skill through role-playing and homework in their real care situations. Program evaluations found a significant decrease in hostility over the period of instruction as well as strong caregiver satisfaction with the instruction.

In summary, research on family caregiving, most of which is provided by women, has been focused on the impact on the caregiver and very little on the learning required to give competent care or by the care recipient to learn self-care. Given the pervasiveness of caregiving activities, both impact on care receivers and caregivers seem like basic issues that should long ago have been understood. Perhaps they would have been if they had been part of the paid economy.

SUMMARY

Information about how women are specifically affected is available for a number of disorders and life roles. It is reasonable to believe that educational efforts could be helpful to women dealing with these health situations.

REFERENCES

Agarwal, A. K., & Shah, A. (1997). Menstrual-linked asthma. *Journal of Asthma, 34,* 539–545.

Barlow, J. H., Williams, B., & Wright, C. C. (1997). Improving arthritis self-management among older adults: 'Just what the doctor didn't order'. *British Journal of Health Psychology, 2,* 175–186.

Berg, M. J. (1997). Status of research on gender differences. *Journal of the American Pharmaceutical Association, MS37,* 43–56.

Berlier, M., Burel, C., Lanteaume, A., Vervloet, D., & Charpin, D. (1997). Sex difference in asthma prevalence. *Allergy, 52,* 871–872.

Bradley, C. (Editor). (1994). *Handbook of psychology & diabetes.* Chur, Switzerland: Harwood Academic Publishers.

Burnside, B., & Hodgins, G. (1992). The role of education in a program to treat depression in older women. *Educational Gerontology, 18,* 483–496.

Candib, L. M. (1995). *Medicine and the family.* New York: Basic Books.

Case, A. M., & Reid, R. L. (1998). Effects of the menstrual cycle on medical disorders. *Archives of Internal Medicine, 158,* 1405–1412.

Cohn, B. A., Cirillo, P. M., Wingard, D. L., Austin, D. F., & Roffers, S. D. (1997). Gender differences in hospitalizations for IDDM among adolescents in California, 1991. *Diabetes Care, 20,* 1677–1639.

Collins, C. E., Given, B. A., & Given, C. W. (1994). Interventions with family caregivers of persons with Alzheimer's disease. *Nursing Clinics of North America, 29,* 195–207.

Conley, V. M., & Burman, M. E. (1997). Informational needs of caregivers of terminal patients in a rural state. *Home Healthcare Nurse, 15,* 808–817.

Cooper, P. J., Coker, S., & Fleming, C. (1994). Self-help for bulimia nervosa: A preliminary report. *International Journal of Eating Disorders, 16,* 401–404.

Cooper, P. J., Coker, S. & Fleming, C. (1996). An evaluation of the efficacy of supervised cognitive behavioral self-help for bulimia nervosa. *Journal of Psychosomatic Research, 40,* 281–287.

Covan, E. K. (1997). Cultural priorities and elder care: The impact on women. *Health Care for Women International, 18,* 329–342.

Droppelman, P. G., Thomas, S. P., & Wilt, D. (1995). Anger in women as an emerging issue in MCH. *Maternal Child Nursing, 20,* 85–94.

Dwyer, K. A. (1997). Psychosocial factors and health status in women with rheumatoid arthritis: Predictive models. *American Journal of Preventive Medicine, 13,* 66–72.

Ferrell, B. R., Ferrell, B. A., Ahn, C. & Tran, K. (1994). Pain management for elderly patients with cancer at home. *Cancer, 74,* 2139–2146.

Ferrell, B. R., Grant, M., Chan, J., Ahn, C., & Ferrell, B. A. (1995). The impact of cancer pain education on family caregivers of elderly patients. *Oncology Nursing Forum, 22,* 1211–1218.

Fields, B., Reesman, K., Robinson, C., Sims, A., Edwards, K., McCall, B., Short, B., Thomas, S. P. (1998). Anger of African American women in the South. *Issues in Mental Health Nursing, 19,* 353–373.

Fitzgerald, J. T., Anderson, R. M., & Davis, W. K. (1995). Gender differences in diabetes attitudes and adherence. *Diabetes Educator, 21,* 523–529.

Frederickson, B. L., & Roberts, T.A. (1997). Objectification theory. *Psychology of Women Quarterly, 21,* 173–206.

Friedman, S. S. (1998). Girls in the 90s: A gender-based model for eating disorder prevention. *Patient Education & Counseling, 33,* 217–224.

Gallagher-Thompson, D., & DeVries, H. M. (1994). "Coping with frustration" classes: Development and preliminary outcomes with women who care for relatives with dementia. *Gerontologist, 34,* 548–552.

Goeppinger, J., & Lorig, K. (1996). Interventions to reduce the impact of chronic disease: Community-based arthritis patient education. In J. J. Fitzpatrick & J. Norbeck (Eds.), *Annual review of nursing research,* Vol. 15, pp. 101–122. New York: Springer Publishing Co.

Gordon, V., & Ledray, L. (1986). Growth-support intervention for the treatment of depression in women of middle years. *Western Journal of Nursing Research, 8,* 263–283.

Harris, R. Z., Benet, L. Z., & Schwartz, J. B. (1995). Gender effects in pharmacokinetics and pharmacodynamics. *Drugs, 50,* 222–239.

Hartman-Stein, P., & Reuter, J. M. (1988). Developmental issues in the treatment of diabetic women. *Psychology of Women Quarterly, 12,* 417–428.

Kenshole, A. (1997). Contraception and the woman with diabetes. *Canadian Journal of Diabetes Care, 21,* 14–18.

Kleffel, D. (1998). Lives on hold. *Home Healthcare Nurse, 16,* 465–472.

Lahita, R. G. (1996). The connective tissue diseases and the overall influence of gender. *International Journal of Fertility, 41,* 156–165.

Legato, M. J. (1997). Gender-specific physiology: How real is it? How important is it? *International Journal of Fertility, 42,* 19–29.

Liporace, J. D. (1997). Women's issues in epilepsy. *Postgraduate Medicine, 102,* 123–138.

Macdonald, J. (1997). Needs assessment for a diabetes and menopause program. *Canadian Journal of Diabetes Care, 21,* 19–24.

Mathias, S. D., Kupperman, M., Liberman, R. F., Lipschutz, R. C., & Steege, J. F. (1996). Chronic pelvic pain: Prevalence, health-related quality of life, and economic correlates. *Obstetrics & Gynecology, 87,* 321–327.

Mazzuca, S. A., Brandt, K. D., Katz, B. P., Chambers, M., Byrd, D., & Hanna, M. (1997). Effects of self-care education on the health status of inner-city patients with osteoarthritis of the knee. *Arthritis & Rheumatism, 40,* 1466–1474.

Meagher, D., & Murray, D. (1997). Depression. *Lancet, 349,* sI17–sI20.

Miaskowski, C. (1997). Women and pain. *Critical Care Nursing Clinics of North America, 9,* 453–458.

Mirowsky, J. (1996). Age and the gender gap in depression. *Journal of Health & Social Behavior, 37,* 362–380.

National Institute of Diabetes and Digestive & Kidney Diseases, National Institutes of Health. (1995). *Diabetes in America* (2nd ed.). Bethesda: Author.

Nattrass, M. (1996). *Malin's clinical diabetes* (2nd ed.). London; Chapman & Hall Medical.

Norcross, W. A., Ramirez, C., & Palinkas, L. A. (1996). The influence of women on the health care-seeking behavior of men. *Journal of Family Practice, 43,* 475–480.

Olmsted, M. P., Davis, R., Rockert, W., Irvine, M. J., Eagle, M., & Garner, D. M. (1991). Efficacy of a brief group psychoeducational intervention for bulimia nervosa. *Behavioral Research & Therapy, 29,* 71–83.

Osborne, M. L., Vollmer, W. M., Linton, K. L. P., & Buist, A. S. (1998). Characteristics of patients with asthma within a large HMO. *American Journal of Respiratory & Critical Care Medicine, 157,* 123–128.

Paterson, B. L., Thorne, S., & Dewis, M. (1998). Adapting to and managing diabetes. *Image, 30,* 57–62.

Polonsky, W. H., Anderson, B. J., Lohrer, P. A., Aponte, J. E., Jacobson, A. M., & Cole, Charlotte F. (1994). Insulin omission in women with IDDM. *Diabetes Care, 17,* 1178–1185.

Prescott, E., Lange, P., Vestbo, J., & The Copenhagen City Heart Study Group. (1997). Effect of gender on hospital admissions for asthma and prevalence of self-reported asthma: A prospective study based on a sample of the general population. *Thorax, 52,* 287–289.

Redman, B. K. (1997). *The practice of patient education (ed. 8).* St. Louis; Mosby-Year Book.

Redman, B. K. (1998). *Measurement tools in patient education.* New York: Springer Publishing Co.

Roberto, K. A. (1994). The study of chronic pain in later life: Where are the women? *Journal of Women & Aging, 6,* 1–7.

Roberto, K. A. (1997). Chronic pain in the lives of older women. *Journal of the American Medical Women's Association, 52,* 127–131.

Schmidt, U., Ali, S., Sloane, G., Tiller, J., & Treasure, J. (1995). The Eating Disorders Awareness Test: A new instrument for the assessment of the effectiveness of psychoeducational approaches to the treatment of eating disorders. *European Eating Disorders Review, 3,* 103–110.

Shaul, M. P. (1995). From early twinges to mastery: The process of adjustment in living with rheumatoid arthritis. *Arthritis Care & Research, 8,* 290–297.

Shaul, M. P. (1997). Transitions in chronic illness: Rheumatoid arthritis in women. *Rehabilitation Nursing, 22,* 199–205.

Smith, C. E. (1996). Quality of life and caregiving in technological home care. *Annual review of nursing research* (Vol. 14, pp. 95–118). New York: Springer Publishing Co.

Sprock, J., & Yoder, C. Y. (1997). Women and depression: An update on the report of the APA task force. *Sex Roles, 36,* 269–303.

Stensland, S. (1998). Resources for the care giver of the person with cancer. *Cancer Practice, 6,* 51–55.

Thiels, C., Schmidt, U., Treasure, J., Garthe, R., & Troop, N. (1998). Guided self-change for bulimia nervosa incorporating use of a self-care manual. *American Journal of Psychiatry, 155,* 947–953.

Thomas, S. P. (1995). Women's anger: Causes, manifestations, and correlates. In C. D. Spielberger and others (Eds.), *Stress and emotion.* New York: Taylor & Francis.

Thomas, S. P. (1997). Women's anger: Relationship to suppression to blood pressure. *Nursing Research, 46,* 324–330.

Thomas, S. P. (1998). Assessing and intervening with anger disorders. *Nursing Clinics of North America, 33,* 121–133.

Tinker, L. F. (1994). Diabetes mellitus—A priority health care issues for women. *Journal of the American Dietetic Association, 94,* 976–985.

Treasure, J., Schmidt, U., Troop, N., Tiller, J., Todd, G., Keilen, M., & Dodge, E. (1994). First step in managing bulimia nervosa: Controlled trial of therapeutic manual. *British Medical Journal, 308,* 686–689.

Troisi, R. J., et. al. (1995). Menopause, postmenopausal estrogen preparations, and the risk of adult-onset asthma. *American Journal of Respiratory & Critical Care Medicine, 152,* 1183–1188.

Tucker, L. F. (1994). Diabetes mellitus—a priority health care issue for women. *Journal of the American Dietetic Association, 94,* 976–985.

Turk, D. C., Okifuji, A. & Scharff, L. (1994). Assessment of older women with chronic pain. *Journal of Women & Aging, 6,* 25–42.

Unruh, A. M. (1996). Gender variations in clinical pain experience. *Pain, 65,* 123–167.

Vallerand, A. H. (1998). Development and testing of the Inventory of Functional Staus—Chronic Pain. *Journal of Pain & Symptom Management, 15,* 125–133.

West, P., & Isenberg, M. (1997). Instrument development: The Mental Health-related Self-care Agency Scale. *Archives of Psychiatric Nursing, 11,* 126–132.

Xie, C. X., Piecoro, L. T., & Wermeling, D. P. (1997). Gender-related considerations in clinical pharmacology and drug therapeutics. *Critical Care Nursing Clinics of North America, 9,* 459–468.

CHAPTER EIGHT

Patient Education for Women: Summary

L ike other forms of education, patient education has been used to reproduce the social order. It is a form of power that in some instances may have been used more to control than to empower, witness the fact that for years its major focus was achieving compliance with the physician's regimen. There are signs that this trend is slowly yielding to a new reality. Assisting patients to make their own decisions, interest in lay models of disease explanation, and teaching self-management that actually incorporates the patient's goals and life pattern are examples of this dawning reality.

The purpose of this final chapter is to explore ethical issues in patient education, as well as learning styles, instructional approaches and goals of patient education for women. In addition, the themes of the book will be summarized.

ETHICAL ISSUES

The practice of patient education for women clearly can do more to be supportive of autonomy for individual women and to be fairer to females as a group. Examples have been provided throughout this book. Although education can support autonomy by empowering women to create and choose options, it can also reinforce oppressive messages and structures. As in all other areas of health care, there is a constant struggle to move from the old provider-centered sets of attitudes and actions, to support informed patient autonomy for women of all cultures, ages, abilities, and classes.

Examples of lack of fairness to groups of women are legion. Women with spinal-cord injuries were twice as likely as men to report having received no sexual education and counseling. Disabled women have also reported difficulty obtaining reliable contraceptive information and find use of various methods difficult because of their disability. Since in the past women with severe physical disabilities were discouraged from having children, there have been few studies of pregnancy among these women. There is also a lack of good quality information about health care needs of these women during menopause or the detection and treatment of sexually transmitted diseases. Although women with disabilities need to receive better education about sexuality issues, a serious prior problem is lack of awareness and sensitivity to these issues on the part of providers (Becker, Stuifbergen, & Tinkle, 1997).

Measurement tools that have been found to show gender bias also can be unfair. A couple of examples will show the problem. One of the most consistent findings in epidemiological studies of depression is the greater prevalence rate of depressive symptoms among women compared to men. It is difficult to say whether these disparities actually reflect higher rates of depressive disorders among women, a greater tendency for women to express their feelings, or whether they are simply an artifact of measurement procedures. Stommel and others (1993) found gender bias in the measurement properties of the Center for Epidemiologic Studies Depression Scale (CES-D). One of the most widely used self-report instruments to measure depressive symptomatology in nonpsychiatric populations, the CES-D Scale, was found to contain two items that showed different response patterns among men and women. Stommel and others (1993) constructed a revised scale that tested free of gender bias with a large sample of persons with cancer and their caregivers.

A second example of gender bias in measurement has been discovered in the Rose Questionnaire Angina (Garber, Carleton, & Heller, 1992). The Rose Questionnaire is commonly used to determine the prevalence of angina pectoris in epidemiologic studies and in clinical trials to assess treatment effects and predict subsequent cardiovascular morbidity and mortality. Measurements from this tool have been found not to differentiate well between patients with and without myocardial ischemia as demonstrated by thallium-201 myocardial scintigraphy, particularly among females. These results suggest that the Rose Questionnaire may be of limited validity for these purposes, especially when used with women. It is likely that many measurement tools have not been checked for gender bias, including those used to assess patients' educational needs and/or to evaluate the effects of patient-education programs.

A final example of lack of fairness lies in assumptions underlying health policies that considerably impact women. The widespread use of emergency postcoital contraception could prevent many unintended pregnancies and abortions each year in the United States. The method is underused because it must be prescribed by a doctor and taken within 72 hours after intercourse; medical consultation is difficult to arrange on such short notice. Although in some countries health ministers have considered making emergency contraception available without a prescription and selling it in pharmacies, it is not yet so available. Many doctors and the public believe that easy access to emergency contraception would encourage promiscuity and unsafe sexual relations and discourage the use of reliable contraception (Glasier & Baird, 1998).

A test of the safety of making this drug available to women at home found that women were able to self-administer it correctly, at the appropriate time and without adverse effects, and did not appear to abandon more reliable methods of contraception (Galsier & Baird, 1998). An obvious question concerning this issue is why public policy about this drug should deny women access to it as opposed to making the drug available to be used by women with full informed consent and teaching so that they will use it correctly.

The obvious question to ask about patient education is whether in its current institutional placement it can play the advocacy role that women need. Can current programs of patient education arm women with the knowledge and skills they need to challenge a system when it is not treating them fairly? No evidence on this point could be found. Clearly, there is a need for such advocacy education for women, which may have to be developed outside the system.

LEARNING STYLES, EDUCATIONAL APPROACHES, AND EFFECTS

In general, the literature on gender differences in learning does not provide much direction for patient education. Learning style is an individual's characteristic way of processing information, feeling, and behaving in learning situations. Philbin, Meier, Huffman, and Boverie (1995) conclude that there are insufficient data to definitively answer questions comparing women's and men's learning styles. The research on causal attributions and perceptions of control has not found consistent differences between males and females. Gender differences in mastery or self-efficacy (SE) are likely to be linked to differences in social experiences. Specifically, a consistently unresponsive or negative environment has been found to affect a person's sense of SE, which in turn leads to anxiety and depression. Studies of coping may not encompass aspects that are of particular importance to women, such as relationship-focused coping (Chesney & Ozer, 1995).

Conclusions from multiple studies of intelligence suggest that females on average score higher on tools that require rapid access to certain kinds of long-term memory, production and comprehension of complex prose, fine-motor skills and perceptual speed. Males on average score higher on tasks that require transformations in visual-spatial work, memory, motor skills involving aiming, and fluid reasoning especially in math and scientific domains (Halpern, 1997).

Review of recent meta-analyses of patient-education studies show no breakout effect by gender, presumably because breakdown of outcome by this variable was not available in most of the original studies. Brown (1992) analyzed 73 studies of the effect of diabetes education and considered age but not gender. Devine (1992a) notes that the large research base of controlled clinical trials on the effects of patient education and psychoeducational care to adult surgical patients shows that patients who received these interventions recovered more quickly, experienced less postsurgical pain, had less psychological distress, and were more satisfied with the care they received than were patients receiving the psycheducational care usually provided in the setting. In this research (187 studies), the beneficial effects of psychoeducational care were found in both males and females in adults of different ages hospitalized for many different types of surgery across the time span of 1960 to 1982.

In an overlapping meta-analysis of 191 studies of the effects of psychoeducational care for adult surgical patients for the time period 1963–1989, Devine (1992b) noted that 68% of studies included both males and females. No analysis of differential learning effects by gender was reported in the meta-analysis. Although the proportion of the original study populations that were female and how representative they were of the general population of females was also not reported, one could tentatively assume that the benefits of educational care to adult surgical patients is available to females.

Meta-analysis of 102 studies from the time period 1965–1993, of the effects of psychoeducational care on blood pressure included some emphasis on ethnicity but no mention of gender (Devine & Reifschneider,

1995). Analysis of 116 studies of psychoeducational care provided to adults with cancer reported that 70% of studies included more women than men with 18% including only women. Psychoeducational care was found to provide benefits related to anxiety, depression, mood, nausea, vomiting, pain, and knowledge. Differentiating among the effectiveness of various types of psychoeducational care was problematic (Devine & Westlake, 1995). Analysis of 45 randomized experimental studies of a variety of psychosocial interventions with adult cancer patients showed effect sizes from the educational interventions of .25 for emotional adjustment, .27 for functional adjustment, .21 for symptoms, and .80 for medical measures including physician rating of disease progression (Meyer & Mark, 1995).

Meta-analysis of 31 studies of the effects of psychoeducational care in adults with asthma, published between 1972 and 1993 showed that both education and relaxation-based behavioral interventions improved important clinical outcomes. In 27 studies gender was reported; 85% of these had more women than men. Treatments providing education alone showed a d_+ value of .35 or larger, with important effects on occurrence of asthmatic attacks, respiratory function, functional status, adherence to treatment regime, and other outcomes. Methodological weaknesses in a number of the studies indicate caution about the stability of the findings (Devine, 1996).

Meta-analysis of 28 controlled studies of cardiac patient education did not report effects by sex, although inspection of the demographic characteristics of subjects in the original research shows that where sex was reported, an average of 85% of subjects were male. Results of the meta-analysis indicate that cardiac patient education programs have demonstrated a measurable impact on blood pressure, mortality, exercise, and diet (Mullen, Mains, & Velez, 1992). In view of the composition of the study samples, generalization to female patients likely remains to be established.

A meta-analysis of 72 studies of teaching strategies for patients apparently did not code the original studies by gender (assuming this variable was described in the study). The meta-analysis showed that structured teaching strategies had the largest effect size, with reinforcement, independent study, and use of multiple teaching strategies also important (Theis & Johnson, 1995). This author is not aware of any other summary work elucidating whether particular teaching strategies are more effective for women than for men and if so which ones. A complete list of meta-analyses and research reviews in patient education may be found in Redman (1997).

GOALS OF PATIENT EDUCATION FOR WOMEN

Feminist and other critiques described throughout this book suggest particular goals for patient education for women, in addition to the more general goals of patient eduction. A list of some of these goals follows.

1. Provide gender-sensitive care, which acknowledges differences in the nature, experience, presentation, risk factors, etiology, and consequences of the health problem in the needs and expectations of men and women regarding health care services, and in their responses to the implications of treatment. Gender-sensitive care takes women's health complaints and experiences seriously and uses their expertise to strengthen self-determination (Gijsbers van Wijk, van Vliet & Kolk, 1996).
2. Promote empowerment—recognizing, promoting, and enhancing women's abilities to meet their own needs, solve their own problems, and mobilize necessary resources to take control of the factors that affect their health. At the same time, it is extremely important not to deflect attention from the structures that perpetuate women's social inequities (Anderson, 1996). Patient education can have a profound effect on how women allow their actual or potential health problems to control their lives and on how they see developing their health potential and its ability to enable them to carry out their life plans. Anderson (1996) provides examples of immigrant women unable to speak the language of the health care provider and how this situation almost assures that clinical misunderstandings persist and the possibilities for treatment negotiation are minimal. People unable to communicate in English have difficulty getting the information they need to manage illness in a way that is acceptable to health professionals and the patient is seen as noncompliant.
3. Identify and change education that enforces socially prescribed limits in a patriarchal society that still may be discriminatory on the basis of gender, ethnic origin, and age.
4. Develop a clear sense of gender fairness in educational services in health. Questions have been raised throughout this text of unequal access to health services and in some instances to educational services, as well as to large bodies of research undergirding health care that do not include sufficient numbers of women to provide equally effective care or educational services for them. Obviously, our society judged these conditions to be fair. Many have now

raised strong objection to these past notions of fairness, which must now be replaced with new norms, which are still under development.

SUMMARY OF THEMES IN THIS BOOK

This book is based on the notion that education can be both empowering to women or can continue to reinforce their subordination. Our professional ethic requires us to advocate for and practice in ways that will best serve our women patients. Our responsibility is to assure that the research necessary to provide them with good care is accomplished and used in direct service, and to honor their sense of autonomy, their informed preferences, and choices. Otherwise, we are complicitous in teaching women culturally biased information and/or in setting expectations for them that are unreachable because social policies do not support them.

Throughout the book, feminist and sociological critiques of educational practices of the health care system have been put forth. Analysis of the educational literature shows a pattern consistent with selective attention to the reproductive aspects of women's health and their societal goals, and far less focus on topics of interest to women themselves for their subjective well-being. An example is the lack of education about how women of all socioeconomic groups move through the menopausal transition.

The following additional themes are noteworthy:

- Whole areas of education for women can be dominated by information biased through commercial interests for products, institutional services, or through unbalanced media coverage. Perhaps slightly more subtle, patient education has generally been focused on a medical agenda as opposed to the agendas of the women involved.
- Almost no literature about gender differences important to patient education for children were found.
- A female propensity for collaboration and conferring with others in their network was found in several studies. In subject areas thought to be private and in some cultures, a taboo against communication with males exists.

- Although most work has been done with White middle-class women with strong levels of formal education, scholarship basic to good educational services for many others groups of women is increasing.
- Some women simply will not accept the limitations of a pure medical model either because it does not fit with their daily lives or because they perceive that medicine has been biased against them in the past as part of a cultural authority not in their best interest.
- Social policies are disadvantaging women in a number of areas: insurance coverage for acute rather than chronic care, concentration of rehabilitation resources in areas that predominantly affect males, recognizing caregiving as a personal rather than a societal responsibility, and so on.
- The educational approach to AIDS prevention can be seen as a case study in putting women in the impossible position of being responsible for men's behavior.
- New genetic technologies fall heavily on women; there is a need for special attention to educational approaches as well as full disclosure, which will support women's autonomy in the decisions that must be made as a result of these tests.
- Lesser access to resources including effective care and educational programs based on their special needs has afflicted women; a case example of this discrimination is cardiovascular care including rehabilitation.
- There is very poor development of educational programs for very common problems and developmental stages for women; menarche, menopause, osteoporosis, urinary incontinence, and mitral valve prolapse are examples.
- It is quite possible that many measurement tools have not been checked for gender bias, making findings from studies using these tools open to question and perhaps misdirecting clinical assessments based on them.

The book also highlights several dilemmas:

- Most comparisons of women's health and learning are with those of men, which perpetuates the notion of a male standard. Perhaps these comparisons are useful to show inequity, which is still being described, but in the long run, the standards of women's health should form a female "gold standard."
- Women experience inequity in provider-patient consultations including diagnostic tests, treatment and rehabilitation, yet women

use more health services. Does this happen, because they do not get satisfactory outcomes from the care or because their conditions, especially those that are reproductive, are so defined by medicine as to require its services?
- Educating women to be better caregivers will encourage social institutions to place more responsibility on them, unless caregiver education is accompanied by a strong move toward policy change.

Patient education for women is an agenda in the making. It is not without its political risks, especially to advocates who are not in powerful organizational positions, because it will change status quo relationships between providers and health care institutions, and their patients and communities. But it must happen. Standards of care including in patient education must incorporate gender. One could even question whether it will be possible to develop programs of patient education for women under the auspices of the medical care system.

A statement of women's patient-education rights would indicate that all women deserve to be educated to their desired level of competence, using their strengths. Commitment to this standard would mean widespread availability of content, measurement tools to assess pre- and posteducational status, methods to accomodate varying literacy levels, educational services that are culturally appropriate, and full access to all health concerns. These services would focus on development of self-efficacy among the women served, use of the woman's goals, reversing historic trends of education for women for the goals of society and family and to fit with health providers' goals and routines.

REFERENCES

Anderson, J. M. (1996). Empowering patients: Issues and strategies. *Social Science & Medicine, 43,* 697–705.

Becker, H., Stuifbergen, A., & Tinkle, M. (1997). Reproductive health care experiences of women with physical disabilities: A qualitative study. *Archives of Physical Medicine & Rehabilitation, 78*(Suppl. 5), S-26–S-33.

Brown, S. A. (1992). Meta-analysis of diabetes patient education research: Variations in intervention effects across studies. *Research in Nursing & Health, 15,* 409–419.

Chesney, M. A., & Ozer, E. M. (1995). Women and health: In search of a paradigm. *Women's Health, 1,* 3–26.

Devine, E. C. (1992a). Effects of psychoeducational care with adult surgical patients: A theory-probing meta-analysis of intervention studies. In T. D. Cook, H. Cooper, D. S. Cordray, L. V. Hartmann, R. J. Hedges, T. A. Light, T. A. Louis, & F. Mostelle (Eds.), *Meta-analysis for explanation: A casebook.* New York: Russell Sage Foundation.

Devine, E. C. (1992b). Effects of psychoeducational care for adult surgical patients: A meta-analysis of 191 studies. *Patient Education & Counseling, 19,* 129–142.

Devine, E. C. (1996). Meta-analysis of the effects of psychoeducational care in adults with asthma. *Research in Nursing & Health, 19,* 367–376.

Devine, E. C., & Reifschneider, E. (1995). A meta-analysis of the effects of psychoeducational care in adults with hypertension. *Nursing Research, 44,* 237–245.

Devine, E. C., & Westlake, S. K. (1995). The effects of psychoeducational care provided to adults with cancer: Meta-analysis of 116 studies. *Oncology Nursing Forum, 22,* 1369–1381.

Garber, C. E., Carleton, R. A., & Heller, G. V. (1992). Comparison of "Rose Questionnaire Angina" to exercise thallium scintigraphy: Different findings in males and females. *Journal of Clinical Epidemiology, 45,* 715–720.

Gijsbers van Wijk, C. M., van Vliet, K. P., & Kolk, A. M. (1996). Gender perspectives and quality of care: Toward appropriate and adequate health care for women. *Social Science & Medicine, 43,* 707–720.

Glasier, A., & Baird, D. (1998). The effects of self-administering emergency contraception. *New England Journal of Medicine, 339,* 1–4.

Halpern, D. F. (1997). Sex differences in intelligence; implications for education. *American Psychologist, 52,* 1091–1102.

Meyer, T. J., & Mark, M. M. (1995). Effects of psychosocial interventions with adult cancer patients: A meta-analysis of randomized experiments. *Health Psychology, 14,* 101–108.

Mullen, P. D., Mains, D. A., & Velez, R. (1992). A meta-analysis of controlled trials of cardiac patient education. *Patient Education & Counseling, 19,* 143–162.

Philbin, M., Meier, E., Huffman, S., & Boverie, P. (1995). A survey of gender and learning styles. *Sex Roles, 32,* 485–494.

Redman, B. K. (1997). *The practice of patient education* (8th ed.). St. Louis: Mosby.

Stommel, M., Given, B. A., Given, C. W., Kalaian, H. A., Schulz, R., & McCorkle, R. (1993). Gender bias in the measurement properties of the Center for Epidemiologic Studies Depression Scale (CES-D). *Psychiatry Research, 49,* 239–250.

Theis, S. L., & Johnson, J. H. (1995). Strategies for teaching patients: A meta-analysis. *Clinical Nurse Specialist, 9,* 100–120.

Index

Springer Publishing Company

Integrating Complementary Health Procedures into Practice

Carolyn Chambers Clark, EdD, RN, ARNP, HNC, FAAN

This is a practical guide to integrating complementary/alternative therapies into a traditional health care practice. It can be used by nurses, physicians, mental health practitioners, physical therapists–any professional who wants to augment or enhance their services or simply understand what their patients may do on their own to help themselves. The first half provides rationale and strategies for making a blend of traditional and nontraditional strategies and practices work. The second half outlines actual therapies most likely to make a successful complement to traditional practice. A perfect companion volume to the *Encyclopedia of Complementary Health Practice.*

Contents: Preface • General Principles • Reasons for Integrating Complementary Health Procedures into Practice • Overcoming Resistance • Scientific Support for Complementary Procedures • The Practitioner-Client Relationship • Guidelines for Choosing the Right Therapy • Evaluating Results • Costs and Insurance Coverage • Marketing a Complementary Practice • How to Integrate Selected Complementary Therapies • A Healing with Diet , Herbs, and Scents • Nutrition / Supplements • Herbs • Aromatherapy • Traditional Healing Systems • Ayurveda • Chinese Health and Healing • Feng Shui • Mind/Body Therapies • Affirmations • Assertiveness Skills • Breathing • Coping Skills Training • Exercise/Movement • Guided Imagery • Hypnosis • Meditation • Relaxation Therapies • Refuting Irrational Ideas • Touch Therapies • Therapeutic Activities • Art Production/Ritual • Journal Writing • Sound/Music Therapy • Appendix: Training Programs, Educational Resources, and Organizations

2000 352pp. (est) 0-8261-1288-9 www.springerpub.com

536 Broadway, New York, NY 10012-3955 • (212) 431-4370 • Fax (212) 941-7842

SP *Springer Publishing Company*

Nurse-Social Worker Collaboration in Managed Care
A Model of Community Case Management
Joellen W. Hawkins, RNC, PhD, FAAN
Nancy W. Veeder, MSW, MBA, PhD
Carole W. Pearce, RNC, PhD

"It is a perfect time for collaborative efforts among providers, patients, families, and communities...(this book) proposes we have a mutual understanding that patients and their families need coaches in their quest to comprehend and use a new and evolving health care system, and that together we are the key to a winning team."
                              –Faye W.Whitney, PhD, RN, FAAN

*"*****!" "The quantity and quality of experts cited and referenced is formidable. This is a well-organized, easy to read, attractive volume...provides a wealth of information for professionals and educators...the need for this volume is self-evident."*
                              –Sharon Maas, PhD, Doody Publishing

This volume presents a model that clearly maps out and differentiates roles and responsibilities for effective nurse-social work case management teams. A team effort in itself, this book is authored by outstanding individuals from both professions. It features the results of thorough interviews with nursing and social work leaders about collaboration, what works, what doesn't, and recommendations for the future.

Contents: Introduction • Revolution and Chaos in American Health Care • The Settlement House Movement • Social Workers and Nurses on Collaboration • The Biopsychosocial Individual and Systems Intervention Model • Finding Common Ground in the Community • A Flexible, Community-Based Approach to Assessment, Diagnosis, and Outcomes Measurement • The Hospital View • The Community View • Physicians Learn New Roles for Managed Care • Getting It Together • Appendix

One of Doody's "250 BEST" Books!
1998 240pp. 0-8261-9830-9 hard $37.95 (outside US $42.80)

536 Broadway, New York, NY 10012-3955 • (212) 431-4370 • Fax (212) 941-7842

⑤ *Springer Publishing Company*

A Total Wellness Program for Women Over 30

Comprehensive Manual with Medical Guidelines for Health Care Professionals

Barbara Kass-Annese, RNCNP, MSN, Consultants
William Parker, MD
Sharon Schnare, RN, FNP, CNM

"An A to Z comprehensive guide for health care professionals and a significant contribution for the treatment of women."
 —**Marie Lugani,** President and Founder of the American Menopause Foundation Inc.

This manual provides a comprehensive wellness program for women in preparation as they age. It blends western conventional medicine with complementary (alternative) health care practices. The total wellness approach includes exercise, nutrion, vitamin and mineral therapy, and stress management as its foundation.

Contents: Acknowledgments • Introduction • From Perimenopause to Postmenopaus • Symptoms of the Climacteric • Cardiovascular Disease • Osteoporosis and Other Health Issues • Psychological, Sociological, and Sexual Issues Associated with the Climacteric • A Total Wellness Program for Women • Hormonal and Drug Therapies • Complementary Therapies, Holistic Medicine; Final Remarks • Guidelines for the Care of Women Over 30 • In Closing • Appendix A • Appendix B • Bibliography and Resources • References • Evaluation Form

1997 429pp. 0-8261-1180-7 softcover www.springerpub.com

536 Broadway, New York, NY 10012-3955 • (212) 431-4370 • Fax (212) 941-7842